Godfrey Devereux has been a student and teacher of yoga for many years. He has travelled widely, both teaching and running courses on yoga. He now works as the principle teacher at The Life Centre in London, and is the only recognized teacher in the UK of a new form of yoga called Dynamic Yoga.

The *Elements of* is a series designed to present high quality introductions to a broad range of essential subjects.

The books are commissioned specifically from experts in their fields. They provide readable and often unique views of the various topics covered, and are therefore of interest both to those who have some knowledge of the subject, as well as to those who are approaching it for the first time.

Many of these concise yet comprehensive books have practical suggestions and exercises which allow personal experience as well as theoretical understanding, and offer a valuable source of information on many important themes.

In the same series

The Aborigine Tradition
Alchemy
The Arthurian Tradition
Astrology
The Bahá'í Faith
Buddhism
Celtic Christianity
The Celtic Tradition
The Chakras
Christian Symbolism
Creation Myth
Dreamwork
The Druid Tradition
Earth Mysteries
Egyptian Wisdom
Feng Shui
Gnosticism
The Goddess
The Grail Tradition
Graphology
Handreading
Herbalism
Hinduism

Human Potential
The I Ching
Islam
Judaism
Meditation
Mysticism
Native American Traditions
Natural Magic
Numerology
Pendulum Dowsing
Prophecy
Psychosynthesis
The Qabalah
Reincarnation
The Runes
Shamanism
Sufism
Tai Chi
Taoism
The Tarot
Visualisation
World Religions
Zen

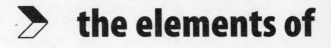

the elements of

yoga
godfrey devereux

Shaftesbury, Dorset •Boston, Massachusetts • Melbourne, Victoria

This book is dedicated to
Reverend T K Holliss for showing me the ocean
Denis Merzel for giving me the compass
Clive Sheridan for pointing out which way the wind blows

© Element Books Limited 1994
Text © Godfrey Devereux 1994

First published in Great Britain in 1994 by
Element Books Limited
Shaftesbury, Dorset SP7 8BP

Published in the USA in 1994 by
Element Books, Inc.
160 North Washington Street, Boston, MA02114

Published in Australia in 1994 by
Element Books
and distributed by Penguin Australia Ltd
487 Maroondah Highway, Ringwood, Victoria 3134

Reprinted 1995

Reprinted 1997
Reprinted June 1997 and January 1998

Cover design by Max Fairbrother
Designed by Roger Lightfoot
Typeset by Footnote Graphics, Warminster, Wiltshire
Printed and bound in Great Britain by
Biddles Ltd, Guildford and King's Lynn

British Library Cataloguing in Publication
Data available

Library of Congress Cataloging in Publication
Data available

ISBN 1–86204–074–5

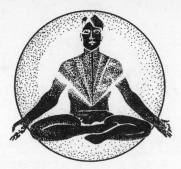

CONTENTS

Introduction   vi

Part 1: What is Yoga?
1. Yoga Defined   3
2. The History of Yoga   8
3. The Philosophy of Yoga   25
4. The Field of Energy and the Subtle Body   33
5. The Limbs of Ashtanga Yoga: 1–5   40
6. The Limbs of Ashtanga Yoga: 6–8   48
7. The Effects of Yoga   62

Part 2: The Practice of Yoga Sadhana
8. General Guidelines   71
9. The Postures, Breathing and Meditation   78

Part 3: Yoga as a Way of Life
10. Yoga and Daily Life   117

Glossary   124
Further Reading   130
Useful Addresses   131
Index   133

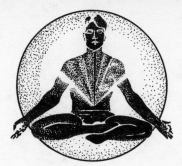

INTRODUCTION

Yoga is a profound, powerful approach to living. As it developed, its methods found their way into Hinduism, Buddhism, Jainism, Islamic Sufism and Contemplative Christianity. The habit of identifying it with Hinduism is mistaken as it is not a religion and does not belong to any. It is, rather, a crucible of spiritual experience from which religions emerge. On a practical level it is a methodology accessing the depths of human nature and penetrating the subtleties of mind and matter. The association between Hinduism and yoga is simply that, historically, most yogis have been Indian and therefore usually Hindu. This, however, is beginning to change: yoga is now more common in the West, particularly Britain and the United States, than in India. Moreover, the most refined development of yoga has occurred over the last thousand years in China and Japan in the form of Zen Buddhism.

The methods of yoga are many and encompass a number of systems, or paths, each with a different emphasis. What makes them yoga is their common purpose, similar effects and shared result. Their purpose is to liberate the individual from unnecessary confusion and pain. Their effect is to generate a quietening and refining of the mind. Their result is peace, joy and happiness in a rich, fulfilling life. In effect yoga is a science of skilful living rather than a religion, it is practical rather than hypothetical. Any philosophical concepts that are related to yoga derive directly from the experiences of yoga. While being mystics and seers, great yogis are also scientists, in that experience that can be repeated at will is the bedrock of their vocation. Although faith in its validity is an essential motivator in yoga, it is not enough to elicit its fruits. Unprejudiced enquiry, rigorous self-discipline and meticulous self-reflection are also necessary.

The beauty of yoga is threefold. One is that it requires, besides the will to practise and a competent guide, nothing other than what we all already have: body, heart and mind. We need no special equipment, building or anything else — just a little space and a little time. The second is that it takes effect immediately one begins to practise and, as one continues, these effects deepen until mind and body are so well disciplined that confusion and sorrow are replaced by a generous happiness that is unmistakable. Third is that anyone can do it and anyone can succeed. It does not depend on any kind of special talent or intelligence or creativity. It is available to anyone, regardless of age, health or mobility, who has the desire to practise and the will to do so consistently. What is more, flexibility, strength and stamina are not particular to any body type: everyone, large or small, overweight or underweight, short or tall can enjoy and benefit from yoga.

Whoever begins yoga and continues regularly and consistently will soon benefit from its fruit. These include suppleness, strength, energy, good posture, improved respiration, circulation and digestion, bright and clear eyes, smooth and shining skin, even muscle tone, normalized body weight, perceptual and verbal clarity, concentration, tranquillity, self-confidence, openness, honesty, temperance, enthusiasm, appreciation and gratitude. It gives one the means and the desire to live life fully, to engage directly with the flavours and textures of life with enthusiasm and joy. However, yoga has a very different curve of progress for each individual. Some people progress physically faster than they progress psychologically, and vice versa. Yoga is more truly about the mind than the body and one should avoid establishing unrealistic goals and mileposts based on what one would like or has seen in others. If it makes you happy about yourself it is working, no matter how much or little flexibility, strength or stamina you develop. These will come with time and practice.

With a pay-off as bounteous as this it is surprising that more people do not practise yoga. To a great extent this is a consequence of the way yoga has been presented, more by academics than by yogis themselves, in the West. This has given it an aura of esoteric mysticism which is an arbitrary emphasis. Yoga is a means for releasing and developing the latent potential of the human body and mind which, when stabilized and harmonized, allow us to live deeper, richer, more creative and satisfying lives. While there *is* a mystical, esoteric side to yoga this is only one emphasis among many, and suited only to people with deep mystical inclinations and to a culture which actively supports a mystical lifestyle. This is not the case in the modern Western world. Those who wish to pursue that approach to yoga should head fast for the Himalayas before it has disappeared even from there, as it has from much of India. But yoga can be, and always has been, used as a way to enrich the lives that we live in the everyday world. It is not a means of escape from, but a passport to, the heart of reality, where we begin to see

A world in a grain of sand,
And a heaven in a wild flower,
Hold infinity in the palm of your hand,
And eternity in an hour

and in that seeing live from a peace and a joy as generous as it is profound.

With grateful acknowledgement to:
Pat Hudson, Phil Powrie, Karin Stephan, Leila Schwartz,
Mira and Shyam Mehta, Narayani, Derek Ireland,
B. K. S. Iyengar, Danny Paradise, B. N. S. Iyengar,
David Swenson, John Scott and all my other teachers
masquerading as my students

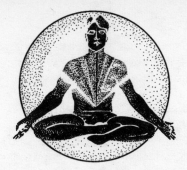

PART 1

WHAT IS YOGA?

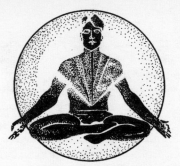

1 · YOGA DEFINED

THE MEANING OF YOGA

The word *yoga* means union. This applies both to the practice and the goal of yoga. By uniting the different aspects of the human body/mind the individual is brought into direct relationship with the flow of reality. This is achieved in different ways, all of which are designed to overcome the habitual sense of isolation that characterizes individual consciousness.

This sense of isolation is replaced by a sense of identity with the vast sweep of reality, which is found to be nothing other than the true nature of the individual. This realization brings about a freedom from the ignorance that is the root cause of human suffering. It therefore brings about liberation: from ignorance, from recurring patterns of suffering, or from the wheel of life and death.

No matter which approach one follows it is important to realize that the methods of yoga are not sacraments. They are simply means to an end which must, though, be constantly reasserted by the means. They are designed to quieten the compulsive activity of the mind and its habit of limited identification with transient aspects of reality; to change our consciousness from one of apartness and separateness to one of identification and union.

In the different systems the state of union is developed

through a different process of gradual unification. The final stages always involve the creation of states of deep inner concentration and absorption, or meditation. In the Bhakti Yoga tradition the process occurs through unifying the energies and inclinations of heart and feeling through ritual devotion. In the Jnana Yoga tradition it is reached by unifying the various tendencies of the mind: memory, reasons, analysis, conceptualization. In the Karma Yoga tradition the emphasis is on unifying the energies of the body and mind through action. In the case of those systems that use the yoga postures – Hatha Yoga, Ashtanga Vinyasa Yoga, Tantra Yoga and Kundalini Yoga – yoga as union applies also on other more tangible levels. Initially there is a unifying of the various aspects of the anatomical body: a restructuring of the musculo-skeletal system. Then, as one goes deeper, there is a harmonizing of the function and relationship between the vital organs of the physiological body. This is followed by a unifying of the body as a whole with the mind, and by the harmonization of the often conflicting tendencies and energies of that mind. In the final stages the process of union becomes more and more similar across the range of yogas.

This process of internalized unification of the various aspects of the human being flowers in the spiritual union of the individual consciousness with the universal reality, or God. The centring of the energies of mind on to very subtle levels harmonizes, resolves and quietens them, bringing about deep inner union. It is then that yoga begins to bear its deepest fruit. Within the quietness that results from a focused mind is revealed the inner quality of human consciousness which is normally hidden. This quality of consciousness is *yoga*, and has many characteristics. They include peace, joy, compassion, discrimination, energy, ease and detachment. When they begin to flower in the consciousness of the practitioner they result in a life that becomes more and more harmonious, joyful and generous.

THE GOAL OF YOGA

Underlying the practice of yoga is an assumption that has been substantiated throughout history by thousands of yogis –

one that can only be verified by applying the techniques, by practising regularly. This is that there is a way of experiencing life that brings great joy, peace and complete fulfilment. It is an experience beyond the power of external forces. It draws upon sources of vitality and strength that ordinarily lie hidden from out perception but that underlie all religious and spiritual endeavour. Some call it knowledge of God, others call it enlightenment. The words are unimportant; the experience is what counts.

No matter what the path, the goal of yoga is the same. No matter what the technique, the effects of yoga are similar. While the ultimate goal, that of self-realization, is obscure for many, there are many flowers that blossom on the path long before that. These include vitality, health, peace of mind, compassion, generosity, understanding and more. The beauty of yoga is that it is a very specific science. It has been developed over millennia and its methodology has been perfected by countless individuals dedicated to its study. It is an exacting science, because its materials are our own minds and bodies. But if we have the motivation and the dedication to pursue the path, the end will be reached.

The goal of yoga has many names, each describing it from a different perspective. Each clarifies the ultimate human condition from a different viewpoint rather than describing a different state:

Yoga means union. As the goal and fruit of yoga it means union of the individual with the universal, the self with other, inner with outer, finite with infinite.

Samadhi refers to the state of consciousness in which liberation is experienced, through extinguishing the movements of the mind caused by desire, confusion and attachment. It is the ultimate state of consciousness, the final fruit of yoga. In it there is neither suffering, nor attachment, nor illusion. There is only the bliss of freedom from limitation and identification of the finite self with the infinite reality.

Moksha means liberation. Often it is thought that yoga is a flight from the world. This is not so. Yoga is a journey into the heart of the world. It is not the world that we leave behind in yoga, but our illusions, our preconceptions about it, especially our deluded sense of our self as separate from God, as apart from all other elements of existence. Free from illusion we become one with the entire universe.

Kaivalya means aloneness. This refers to the fact that when one has become one with God, one with the whole of existence, there is no other, and so one is all alone. This does not imply solitude or loneliness. In it the singular interconnectedness of all is realized.

THE EFFECT OF YOGA

Unfortunately the goal of yoga has been tainted with the brush of fantasy. Many hope the state of *samadhi, moksha* or *kaivalya* is one that will relieve them of stress and bring them to a perfect paradise distinct from the world in which we, ordinary mortals, live. In this state of paradise they believe they will find themselves enjoying a perfection of human character and a sublime transcendental experience. They hope for an end to loneliness, a freedom from desire, the flowering of perfect wisdom, peace and love untainted by the disturbance of human emotion.

Yoga does not turn us into gods. The limitations and troubles of being human cannot be removed but they can be accepted so fully that the flowering of the rich potentiality of the whole human being makes them peripheral to our life. The self-knowledge and equanimity that arise from yoga allow us to develop a more creative relationship with our emotions. Anger, for example, is a perfectly valid human emotion, one that can only be eradicated by becoming cold and insensitive to life. Most people have known the fire of righteous anger: perhaps at the sight of thousands of Ethiopian children dying of starvation in a world which has the resources to adequately feed us all; or upon realizing that environmental degeneration has reached such a critical state that life on earth is at risk.

Yoga does not make us immune to such feelings but it does allow us to process and express our feelings more creatively, positively and responsibly. So we learn to identify strong, habitually destructive emotions as simply waves breaking through our minds. We learn to let go of the habit of identifying our selves with our passing feelings and states of mind. Thus when strong feelings of fear, sadness or anger arise we simply accept and experience them. We do not repress them and make them into a source of unconscious conflict nor do we automatically express them in reactive behaviour patterns. We take responsibility for them by directing out attention to them so completely that they are able to pass as naturally as they arose. They pass because we do not hold on to them and because in directing our attention to them we see into the broader context from which they arise. We see how much of their energy is due to the narrow, grasping action of our mind reacting too quickly to be able to keep a balanced, broad perspective on events and our responses to them. In seeing this we defuse the energy of destructive, reactive responses quite naturally. The negative energy they contained is then made available for the creative process of our lives.

So, while yoga does bring about a purification of character and the cultivation of wisdom, it does not make us super-human. It does not make us immune to life. Instead we learn to live life more skilfully, to take responsibility for our actions, emotions, and for our thoughts. And we learn how that enables us to live more harmoniously with mankind and other forms of life. However, it is vital to realize that the cultivation of wisdom and virtue is gradual, subtle and cannot be forced. They arise through one agency only – that of insight into the real nature of things. They cannot and do not arise just because we want them to. They cannot be put on like a new set of clothes. Only as insight into the impermanence, indivisibility and infinite nature of all phenomena develops through the cultivation of stability and tranquillity do we release those patterns of response that masked our inherent wisdom and virtue. It is useless to pretend to virtue and wisdom. In fact if we act out patterns of behaviour that we think consistent with an image of perfection, wisdom and purity then we plunge ourselves deeper into an inner conflict of ignorance and self-deception.

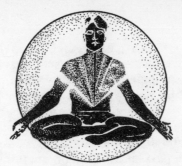

2 · THE HISTORY OF YOGA

The history of yoga can be seen as a record of the different ways that these processes have been developed over five thousand years. Significant archaeological remains, found in 1922 at Mohenjo Daro in the Indus valley, included seals depicting men, or gods, in yogic postures meditating. These seals indicate that the practice of yoga was already significant enough four thousand years ago to have been portrayed artistically. This would not be the case with something that was in its infancy or marginal to the cultural life of those times. How long it had existed before this is open to conjecture, but could as easily be a matter of thousands of years as of hundreds.

The Vedas, the Upanishads, the Bhagavad Gita, the Yoga Sutras and the Yoga Tantras, and a handful of texts concerning Hatha Yoga, constitute the main literature of yoga, to which there is a huge peripheral accumulation. These texts span a period of almost four thousand years up to the eighteenth century. With the works of Sri Aurobindo, Sivananda, Satyananda, B.K.S. Iyengar and others, the literary tradition of yoga is not only ancient, but very much alive. However, the two most important texts are the Bhagavad Gita and the Yoga Sutras. Both contain references to the whole range of yoga techniques and systems but have a different emphasis. The former leans heavily towards the yoga of devotion and selfless action, while the latter leans towards self-reflection and meditation.

However, it is unlikely that in any of these cases the written record marks the origins of the system. It is far more likely that the earliest written descriptions are of methods that had previously been tried and tested within an oral tradition. Given the continuity of the oral tradition in India to the present from ancient times this is a fairly safe assumption and one that is substantiated in a number of ways. One is from the archaeological record which preserves evidence of, for example, meditation taking place at least a thousand years before any written evidence and 2500 years before any comprehensive written systematization of meditation was recorded. Another is from examination of the use of syntax in the written records. Ashtanga Vinyasa Yoga, for example, is described on palm leaves that are about 1500 years old. But the structure of the language in which it is described, and its relationship to the development of sanskrit, suggest that it originated about 3500 years before it was written on the leaves.

Patanjali is often regarded as the father of yoga. However, the Hindu god Siva is traditionally regarded as the source of esoteric yogic knowledge. Many of the tantras, agamas and other works begin by stating that the information contained within was given by Siva to his consort Parvati. In one instance he was overheard by the king of the fishes, Matsyendra, who subsequently took on human form and became the founder of Hatha Yoga. The popular Hindu god Krishna is the source of yogic teachings in the Bhagavad Gita, referring especially to the paths of devotion and action.

CLASSIC YOGA TEXTS

THE VEDAS

Although not specifically yogic texts the Vedas are the earliest written record that include reference to yogic activities. They constitute the oldest existing Hindu literature and include four collections of hymns and rituals composed by mystical seers as a result of their meditative experiences. The oldest is the Rig Veda, from about 1550 BC. It is the first known record of the practice of meditation and its effects. The Arthava Veda also contains specific reference to yogic techniques, including breath control. The other two are the Sama Veda and the Yajur Veda. They are regarded as the divinely inspired source of Hinduism.

THE UPANISHADS

The Upanishads span an era from 900 BC to the twentieth century. They constitute a collection of mystical revelations regarding the nature of reality, human nature and the process of liberation from the bondage of ignorance. They are a significant departure from the ritualistic, institutional literature of the Vedas and are essentially more yogic in spirit. However, it was not until the Middle Ages, mainly the fourteenth and fifteenth centuries, that specific Yoga Upanishads were composed which outline the techniques and effects of specific aspects of Hatha and Kundalini Yoga in particular.

THE BHAGAVAD GITA

Probably composed about 350 BC, the Bhagavad Gita is the most popular and famous work of Yogic and Hindu literature. Many people in India today can recite its entire length of 700 stanzas. Unlike the Upanishads the Gita embraces a yogic approach that does not involve renunciation of worldly action. In it the god Krishna convinces the Prince Arjuna that he must fight a great battle against many relatives in order to fulfil his worldly duty. He goes on to explain a yogic path whereby, by devotion to him (Bakhti Yoga), the meditative process of discernment (Jnana Yoga) and renunciation of the fruits of one's actions (Karma Yoga), one can attain liberation.

THE YOGA SUTRAS

Probably composed about 150 AD (although some scholars place it earlier) by the sage Patanjali, the Yoga Sutras are the major work of esoteric yoga. It describes the nature of human consciousness, the means to overcome its conditioned limitations, and the fruits of liberation in terms of special states of consciousness and special powers. Most great modern yogis acknowledge it as the source point of their lineage. It contains four sections: the first on the state of ecstasy; the second on the path itself; the third on the powers attained on the path, and the fourth on the final fruit of the path: liberation. It describes the eight limbs (ashta anga) of yogic practice and the three-fold basis of yogic action (zeal, self-study and surrender). While the term is not used in the text itself, later commentators have described the yoga system of the Yoga Sutras as Raja Yoga, the royal yoga. The work itself is often referred to as The Yoga Darshana. The greatest emphasis is on developing powerful meditative states.

THE YOGA UPANISHADS

These were composed after the Yoga Sutras, and include the Yoga-Tattva-Upanishad, the Yoga-Raja-Upanishad, the Yoga-Sikkha-Upanishad, the Amrita-Bindu-Upanishad, the Amrita-Nada-Upanishad, the Dhayana-Bindu-Upanishad and others. Together they contain a broad, and often detailed, description of the methods of yoga and their effects, and are written as teachings given by sages or gods to spiritual seekers. The yoga to which they refer is essentially mystical and ascetic and is the practice of renunciates.

THE YOGA TANTRAS

Similar to the Yoga Upanishads are a collection of manuals describing the beliefs, rituals and practices of Tantric Yoga. However they focus more closely on the techniques of awakening the shakti power of the kundalini. This involves physical and psychic concentration techniques that awaken and energize the spiritual channel inside the spinal column. They also include detailed descriptions of the subtle energy body, the chakras (energy centres) and nadis (channels of energy throughout the body). They also claim that in this age of materialistic delusion Tantric Yoga is the only yoga powerful enough to awaken us from the thrall of our delusion.

THE HATHA YOGA PRADIPIKA

Of the many texts specific to Hatha Yoga this is perhaps the most respected. Composed in 1350 AD by Svatmarama, it outlines the practices of Hatha Yoga. In the very first paragraph he defines Hatha Yoga as the stairway to Raja Yoga. Later on he states that perfection in Hatha Yoga cannot be achieved without perfection in Raja Yoga, and vice versa. The text is divided into four sections: the first focuses mainly on the postures; the second on breathing techniques, or pranayama; the third on the locks and seals that are used along with pranayama to awaken the transforming power of the kundalini, which rising from the base of the spine travels upwards energizing and harmonising the energy centres of the subtle body; the fourth on the fruits of yoga. It outlines seven limbs of yoga practice: purification, posture, gestures, internalization, breath control, contemplation, ecstasy.

THE GHERANDHA SAMHITA

Written in the seventeenth century this is one of the major sources of Hatha Yoga instruction. It also outlines seven limbs of yoga practice: purification, posture, gestures, internalization, breath control, contemplation, ecstasy. It begins by stating that Hatha Yoga is the means to ascend the heights of Raja Yoga.

THE SIVA SAMHITA

Written around the turn of the seventeenth century, as in the previous two Hatha Yoga texts a whole section is devoted to the subtle locks and seals that are used to awaken the sleeping kundalini force. These inner techniques are not referred to in other works such as the Vedas, early Upanishads, Bhagavad Gita and Yoga Sutras. They are characteristic of the tantric approach to yoga, which spawned both Hatha and Kundalini

Yoga. This is a body-positive approach whereby the subtle energies of the body are used as the means to awakening and liberation, rather than the subtle dimensions of consciousness.

THE DIVERSITY OF YOGA TODAY

A wide and sometimes confusing array of techniques have been developed which contribute to the process of yoga. These techniques have been emphasized and combined in different ways to make up the different paths of yoga. The way yoga is now taught in the West, with the notable exception of Ashtanga Vinyasa Yoga, rarely reflects accurately any of these historical combinations and therefore can only be inaccurately described as any of the traditional paths of yoga. This, however, does not make them invalid. The range and scope of yoga is vast; its potency profound. Although the ultimate heights of yogic achievement may only be reached by diligent practice of the traditional ways, any partial but sincere practice will result in benefits which are profound and rewarding.

Two examples will clarify this point. Most people who practise the postures of yoga describe their practice as Hatha Yoga. However, they tend not to practise the other limbs of Hatha Yoga nor do they reach proficiency in the key practice of Hatha Yoga, breath control through the use of locks and seals to stabilize and control prana (see pp. 36–7). In effect they are not truly practising Hatha Yoga, for the emphasis and combination of practices are not the traditional ones. Again, many who practise meditation believe that they are practising Raja Yoga. But in the simple manner of the way they hold their body while meditating they often overlook the principle of asana (see pp. 43–5), which is basic to the practice of meditation in Raja Yoga. In the first case, practising yoga postures without the supporting techniques will give little other than purely physical benefit, barely skimming the surface of the fruits of Hatha Yoga. In the second case, observing the mind without stabilizing the body and regulating the breath will calm the mind, but it will not focus the consciousness enough to reach the higher peaks of meditation.

In effect there are emerging in the modern, industrial world new, secular forms of yoga. These approaches to yoga have one powerful benefit that cannot be derived from the traditional ways. They do not require renunciation of our modern, technological lifestyle. Consequently, the transformative effects of their practice remain within the melting pot of society and bring their influence to bear upon it. Yoga has never been exclusively a practice for renunciates. There has always been a householder tradition, wherein practitioners can benefit from the higher powers of body and mind released by yoga without dedicating their lives to it twenty-four hours a day, as was the case with those whose yoga practice was shaped by the great classic texts such as the Yoga Sutras and the Hatha Yoga Pradipika.

The most common elements of traditional yoga techniques taught and practised in the West are the postures, breath control and meditation. Although these are presented as elements of Hatha Yoga, they also belong to other systems, including Ashtanga, Tantra, Kundalini and Ashtanga Vinyasa Yoga. Divorced from the other elements of each of these paths they constitute a new, partial yoga that – although powerful for enriching personal wellbeing – will not bring about the more subtle fruits of practice. These subtle, potent fruits require that the more tangible and accessible elements of yoga be practised in conjunction with the more subtle and potent techniques.

THE UNITY OF YOGA

Each method of yoga uses a different aspect of human consciousness as a lens through which to focus, blend and intensify the overall energy of human consciousness. They also use a different combination of techniques to harness that particular aspect of human consciousness. But often the difference is more on the emphasis placed on the specific techniques than a difference in the techniques themselves. As the effect of practising the techniques deepens the differentiation between them becomes even less clear.

To try to make a neat and precise categorization of yoga techniques into distinct and separate schools which do not

overlap is an expression of the very mentality that yoga liberates us from. Yoga methodology, like reality itself, cannot be
reduced to a simple linear arrangement without repetition,
contradiction and confusion, for yoga is an empirical reality,
not a neat theoretical construct. It fits precisely the unpredictable, paradoxical nature of reality, releasing us from the
linear, sequential either/or mentality of the rational mind.

Any path of yoga undertaken with sincerity will eventually
elucidate the wisdom of Jnana Yoga, inspire the awe and
devotion of Bhakti Yoga, encourage the selfless service of
Karma Yoga, instil the deep tranquillity of Raja Yoga, establish the stability and power of Hatha Yoga, and release the
sexual/spiritual energy (kundalini) of Tantra Yoga. Nurturing
these will be a quality of attention in the yogi that embraces
deep concentration, openness and clarity of mind, calmness
and vitality. So, at a certain point, through the inherent process of unification involved, the methods of yoga unite and
become one. Their differences are simply ones of emphasis
and exist so as to make yoga accessible to every kind of tem-
perament and inclination.

THE PATHS OF YOGA

JNANA YOGA

Jnana Yoga is the yoga of wisdom. It is the Yoga of the Vedas
and the early Upanishads, wherein the real and the unreal are
distinguished by the light of wisdom, through the process of
contemplative meditation. By way of inner enquiry the Jnanin
cultivates the eye of wisdom that reveals the ignorance that
blinds and binds us and the truth that liberates us. Two of the
greatest mystics of modern India Ramakrishna and Ramana
Maharshi, can be regarded as Jnana Yogins, as can Krishnamurti. Jnana Yoga, like Raja Yoga, deeply explores the subtleties of the human mind but, unlike Raja Yoga, in Jnana Yoga
the enquiring spirit of the rational mind is employed. A question is examined and probed until the reasoning and cognitive
faculties of the mind exhaust all its possibilities. An example
is the question 'Who am I?' When reason exhausts itself and

can offer no more answers, the mind, now intensely focused within itself, with no external support, undergoes a climactic shift into the void left by the failure of cogitation. Into this void flowers the awareness of the real that lies behind and beyond the compulsive activity of the mind, however lucid and sophisticated it may be.

TANTRA YOGA

Tantra Yoga is referred to in the yoga tantras as being the only path that can lead to liberation in the current age of Kali Yuga, which is characterized by the destructive effects of selfish desire. Tantra works because it harnesses the basic energy of everyday life and uses it to transform consciousness: the energy of desire. Because this energy is so powerful its application is hazardous, but the risks are necessary as the inertia of this age is otherwise too stagnant for progress to be made in other forms of yoga. The transformation of desire into spiritual ecstasy has always had two paths. On the outer, left-hand path the most extreme and misunderstood form of tantric practice is ritualized sexual intercourse. In this the polarized nature of energy is resolved through conscious, detached sexual activity. It only resembles conventional sexuality outwardly; inwardly it is a totally different experience in which sexual pleasure and desire are used to heighten and clarify awareness. On the inner, right-hand path this energetic resolution and heightening of awareness occurs within the consciousness of the yogin through the use of asana, pranayama and powerful meditative visualizations. All yoga systems that employ and honour the physical body and its energies, especially those emphasizing asana and pranayama (see pp. 43–6), can be said to bear the mark of tantrism. For it is the tantric orientation that states and proves that mind and matter are one, that body and spirit are not separate and that samsara and nirvana – or bondage and liberation – are not two distinct categories of reality. Accordingly both Hatha Yoga (see below) and Kundalini Yoga (a form of yoga awakening the sexual/spiritual energy of the kundalini from the base of the spine) can be categorized as forms of tantric yoga. The experience of the subtle body in asana and pranayama is one in which the heightened awareness and resolution of polarity occurs spontaneously through the balancing of the male and female energies within, ida and pingala (see p. 38).

ASHTANGA VINYASA YOGA

Rediscovered in 1930 by the late Krishnamacharya, this ancient yoga system was recorded on palm leaves 1500 years ago. Its syntax suggests that its oral tradition goes back 5000 years. It is a system that involves intense practice of four series of asana with the aid of pranayama, mudra, bandha and drushti to bring about deep meditation (see chapters 5–7). In it asana involves the simultaneous practice of the other seven limbs of Ashtanga Yoga. There are hundreds of asana in this system. They are given in specific sequences, each designed to harmonize different levels of the body/mind.

The first series restructures the anatomical body, or *annamayakosha*; the second series awakens the pranic body, or *pranamayakosha*; the third series awakens the psychic body, or *manomayakosha*; the fourth series awakens the awareness body, or *vijnanamayakosha*. Having awakened the four outer bodies they all become integrated with the fifth or causal body, *anandamayakosha*, uniting the individual with the absolute.

Bridging the divide between physical (hatha) and mental (raja) yoga, Ashtanga Vinyasa Yoga expresses in a practical way the unity of yoga. Vinyasa means 'setting out and returning', and describes the process of connectivity and synthesis in the practice of yoga. On the most immediate level this is found in the threading together of individual postures into a flowing sequence in which postures are connected by the flowing action of the vinyasa. The vinyasa is a short sequence of postures executed in quick succession following the inbreath and outbreath. A key to the practice is to use a number of locks that help to concentrate the mind and the subtle energies of the body, especially mula bandha (see pp. 54–5), which is also vital to Hatha Yoga pranayama.

ASHTANGA YOGA

The historical father of yoga is generally considered to be Patanjali, the author of the Yoga Sutras. This is a compilation of 196 aphorisms, divided into four sections. In it Patanjali defines the prerequisites, process and effects of yoga, along with a comprehensive analysis of the nature of human consciousness. While the main emphasis of the Yoga Sutras is on meditation, Patanjali presents a methodology involving eight (*ashta*) distinct limbs (*anga*). These limbs are *yama* or moral restraint, *niyama* or observances, *asana* or posture, *pranayama* or breath control, *pratyahara* or internalization, *dharana* or concentration, *dhayana* or absorption, and *samadhi* or transcendence (see chapters 5–6). While these limbs cannot in effect be separated, the last three are referred to as the inner practices, and together constitute the practice of meditation. However, in Ashtanga Yoga, Patanjali makes quite clear that meditation must be supported by the practice of the other limbs. No specific technical instruction is given. This is not because Ashtanga Yoga is theoretical but is rather a perfect example of the way that yoga has been transmitted, with much of the necessarily case-specific practical information being transmitted orally. To write an exhaustive treatise on the numerous asana and pranayama techniques, and how they can be adapted to and applied by different individuals, would be impractical. The power of Patanjali's work is that it contains the seeds of all yoga systems within it. Karma Yoga can be seen as a focused development of *tapas* (zeal), or the effect of yama, niyama, asana and pranayama; Jnana Yoga as that of *svadhyaya* (self study), or the effect of pratyahara and dhayana; Bhakti Yoga as that of *ishvara pranidana* (devotion to the divine), or the effect of dhayana and samadhi; Raja Yoga as a development of dhayana; and Hatha Yoga as that of pranayama. It is easy to see why Ashtanga Yoga as outlined by Patanjali is regarded as the seminal work on yoga.

RAJA YOGA

Raja Yoga, the royal yoga, focuses on the meditation techniques outlined in the Yoga Sutras. While it is referred to in many yoga texts, the Yoga Sutras themselves do not use the term 'raja yoga'. Raja Yoga is understood today as meditation, without reference to the practice of the other limbs of yoga. This has led some Raja yogins to dismiss the postural practices of asana as being superfluous or less spiritual. However this dismissal does not honour the unity or comprehensiveness of yoga. In the Bhagavad Gita the posture for meditation is precisely described in a way that categorizes it as asana. Meditation cannot be experienced without good posture, or calm smooth breathing, or internalization of awareness. If the body loses its stability, the mind will wander and the breath become erratic; when the mind wanders, the body loses its stability and the breath becomes inconsistent. If the breath is erratic, the mind is disturbed and posture collapses. So we find that posture, breath and awareness are the thread that unites each part of our practice, which leads from the more concrete aspect of posture to the more subtle aspect of pure awareness. Raja Yoga is the final flight on the stairway of Ashtanga Yoga: it must be prepared for with Hatha Yoga. It harnesses the subtle energies of consciousness in order to foster awakening and liberation. Its techniques are defined in a number of Yoga Upanishads, including: Yoga-Tattva-Upanishad, Yoga-Shikha-Upanishad, Amrita-Bindu-Upanishad, Amrita-Nada-Upanishad.

HATHA YOGA

Hatha means the will, Hatha Yoga the forceful yoga. Hatha also means sun/moon or male/female; implying the union of complementary but opposite tendencies within the body/mind. While most people assume that posture yoga is Hatha Yoga this is not so. While asana do have a place in Hatha Yoga, the Hatha Yoga texts, such as the Hatha Yoga Pradipika, the Siva Samhita and the Gheranda Samhita, place greater emphasis on the practice of pranayama and the accompanying bandhas. These esoteric techniques cultivate and develop the subtle body. By harnessing the sun and moon currents that flow through the two nostrils the nadis are cleansed and prana stabilized. After stabilizing the subtle body, kundalini can be awakened and directed up the central spiritual channel through the chakras (see pp. 36–9 on the subtle body). The end result is to create a 'divine' body that is so harmonious and potent that it is immune to the effects of time and disease. By cultivating, controlling and stabilizing prana, the yogi's consciousness is also stabilized. At the same time, however, various psychic powers develop, known as the *siddhis*. These powers, including telepathy, are regarded by Raja yogins as dangerous distractions from the essential purpose of yoga. In effect traditional Hatha Yoga was a modern development that was used as a stepping stone to the more subtle meditative techniques of Raja Yoga; it was not seen as something separate from it. Rather it is an emphasis on the aspects of Ashtanga Yoga that involved manipulation of the subtle energy systems of the body made possible through the breathing techniques of pranayama. Mastery of these techniques, combined with mastery of asana, gives the yogin the stability and tranquillity necessary to explore the challenging subtleties of meditation, known as Raja Yoga. In the Hatha Yoga Pradipika, the Gheranda Samhita and the Siva Samhita seven limbs are given to Hatha Yoga. Yama, niyama and dharana are omitted, and the shat kriyas and mudras (including the bandhas) are included. This gives Hatha Yoga a more body-oriented emphasis than Raja Yoga. It harnesses the subtle energies of the body – prana, kundalini and the chakras – to promote awakening and liberation.

BHAKTI YOGA

Bhakti Yoga utilizes the energy of emotions: desire, affection, devotion, love. However, the object of these feelings must be divine, not mortal. Through rituals – including song, dance and mantra – the longing of the human heart for self-transcendence is channelled, intensified and used to loosen the habitual sense of separation that leads automatically to desire, attachment and suffering. There are many strands of Bhakti Yoga, worshipping different gods: Vishnu, worshipped by Vishnaivites, Siva, worshipped by Shaivites, and Krishna. The International Society for Krishna Consciousness is a modern Bhakti movement that has ancient origins. Followers of this movement claim that it is the fastest, easiest and safest way to achieve liberation. The transition required from conventional emotional activity to spiritual application of emotional power is a subtle shift of orientation that requires, at least initially, no demanding exploration of more subtle aspects of human intelligence. In order to utilize the energy of devotion it must be focused, channelled and directed. The higher stages of Bhakti Yoga begin to resemble those of other yogas in the changes in the consciousness of the yogin. While the lens which he uses may be different to focus his energies on to a seed which may be quite specific, the inner process must culminate in samadhi, preceded by dhayana and dharana, as in Ashtanga Yoga and Raja Yoga.

KARMA YOGA

The Bhagavad Gita is the authoritative source for Karma Yoga. The Karma yogin approaches liberation with an attitude to himself and his activities that is self-transcending. This means that whatever his duties, obligations and activities they are undertaken as an offering to the divine, as selfless service: they are not undertaken with regard to their fruits, whether financial, social or even spiritual. By dedicating the fruits of their activity to the divine, Karma yogins are able, through the mundane activity of everyday life, to loosen the bonds of attachment that blind them to their relationship with the absolute. Two well-known Karma yogins are Mahatma Gandhi and Mother Teresa. While it requires no special techniques nor esoteric skills, the method of Karma Yoga is far from easy. It requires considerable commitment and willpower to invest in everyday activities a genuine selflessness. It is not surprising then that the authoritative text for this yoga is also one in which Bhakti Yoga is also emphasized. Giving up the fruits of one's actions becomes more meaningful when there is some higher entity to whom to dedicate them. Again, Karma Yoga cannot be separated from the heightened states of consciousness known as samadhi. Although there are many levels of samadhi, whenever the energies of the body/mind become deeply focused for a sustained period they will arise. This is as true when the lens through which the body/mind focuses is selfless activity as it is to devotion or the subtle movements of consciousness.

MANTRA YOGA

Mantras (see p. 60) have been a part of the repository of yoga for millennia. In many texts their use as a self-contained methodology is referred to as a form of yoga suited to those whose devotion and application is weak. It is not, therefore, regarded as a major yoga. However, as Transcendental Meditation, it has become very well known in the West. Popular ideas about yoga are often based on a superficial view of the role of mantras in yoga. In Mantra Yoga, a short phrase is repeated either audibly or silently to focus and concentrate the mind. Traditionally, the mantra would have a specific spiritual meaning and vibration. This would result in each mantra having a different spiritual effect on the practitioner's consciousness.

MODERN DEVELOPMENTS

There are four contemporary Indian yoga masters whose teachings have spread widely in the West with an initial emphasis on the yoga postures and breathing techniques. Three out of four were students of Krishnamacharya and regard themselves as teaching, in the spirit of Patanjali, Ashtanga Yoga. Of these three, two – B. K. S. Iyengar and Desikachar – have developed their own distinctive approach to yoga postures. The third is Pattabhi Jois, who teaches the classic Ashtanga Vinyasa Yoga, presented in six series rather than the original four. Sivananda, the only one not a direct student of Krishnamacharya, while incorporating the yoga postures into his system placed more emphasis on the relaxing effects of breathing and meditation techniques, within a broad approach to yoga that includes elements of Bhakti, Karma, Hatha and Raja Yoga.

The late Sri Prabupada, the founder of the International

Society for Krishna Consciousness, is another contemporary yoga master who has generated wide interest in the Bhakti Yoga tradition. Sai Baba is another whose yoga leans heavily towards Karma Yoga. There have also been a number of modern yogis exemplifying the Jnana Yoga tradition, including Krishnamurti and Ramana Maharshi.

Iyengar Yoga

Perhaps the most famous, and certainly the most widely followed, modern yogi is B. K. S. Iyengar. Observed in practice by Sivananda he declared that it was like seeing the great Yogi Matsyendra reborn. His approach is unique but not without its critics. It is a direct adaptation of the yoga he was taught by his guru, Krishnamacharya, which is Ashtanga Vinyasa Yoga. In order to make it more accessible, and to allow for individualized therapeutic application, the traditional sequences and dynamic element have been superseded. While Iyengar does occasionally teach a fluid, dynamic approach to asana, which he calls 'jumping', he tends to teach the postures separately. His own practice, however, while not adhering to the traditional sequences does maintain their fluidity and dynamic grace. Iyengar Yoga is a powerful, safe approach to asana and pranayama, taught within the philosophical framework of Patanajali's Yoga Sutras. Although greatly misunderstood by those who have not experienced him, or who are not yet ready for the intensity of his presence, understanding and teaching powers, his emphasis on anatomical alignment paradoxically illuminates the inherent meditative nature of the physical postures. To experience asana through the rigorous application of evenly distributed attention is to discover the interpenetration of mind and body and the meaning of the phrase 'meditation in action'.

Sivananda Yoga

Swami Sivananda was one of the great modern yogis. He wrote many books and inspired many followers. His yoga was brought to the West by Swami Vishnudevananda, and there are now Sivananda centres and ashrams all over the world. Sivananda Yoga emphasizes the five principles of right exercise (asana), right breathing (pranayama), right relaxation, right thinking, and right diet (vegetarian). He summarized yoga as: serve, love, give, purify, meditate, realize. His approach is synchronistic, or holistic, in which the unity and compatibility of the different yoga paths is clarified. It involves the asana and pranayama practices of Hatha Yoga, the devotion of Bhakti Yoga, the mediation of Raja Yoga and the selfless service of Karma Yoga.

Vinniyoga

Developed by T. K. V. Desikachar, son of Krishnamacharya, Vinniyoga is an offshoot of Ashtanga Vinyasa Yoga. In it the asana and pranayama practices are strung together into individually tailored sequences that suit the specific requirements of a given individual at a given moment. The principles of connectivity, fluidity, preparation, counterpoise and breath/body co-ordination are all hallmarks of this method.

Kriya Yoga

Parahamsa Yogananda, author of the *Autobiography of a Yogi*, was one of the first great yogis to come to the West. He taught a method he called Kriya Yoga, which is said to have originated from the almost mythical yogi Babaji, who apparently lived for centuries in the Himalayas in the body of a seventeen-year-old. Kriya Yoga involves the use of special breathing and meditation techniques.

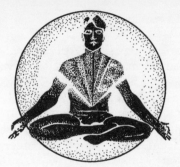

3 · THE PHILOSOPHY OF YOGA

The philosophy of yoga is not speculative. It is the world view that results from practising yoga techniques. Interestingly, it is also a world view that coincides more and more with that of nuclear and quantum physics (see pp. 33–4). While the philosophy of yoga is a vast subject, some vital concepts must be understood in order to gain any insight into the art and science of yoga.

KARMA AND THE WHEEL OF LIFE

In its simplest form karma means the process of action and reaction, whereby one thing leads on, endlessly, to another. It is a concept not unique to India. Jesus of Nazareth declared 'as you sow, so shall you reap'.

Often karma is used as a synonym for fate or destiny. This is not strictly accurate since destiny implies a lack of free will whereas karma very much involves the activity of human will, of intention. Both the physical action and the mental intention create their own reaction. In fact it is the psychological component that is the most vital. The key to karma is how we respond to life. If we respond with skill, we create good karma; if we respond with poor judgement, we create bad karma. Good karma manifests as advantages that life offers us, while bad karma manifests as difficulties. However, good karma can easily turn sour if we react blindly to our good fortune. Equally, bad karma can generate positive opportunities if we apply clarity to the way in which we meet difficulty.

So, the circumstances of life that we meet are the result of past actions. As such they are unavoidable and not subject to our free will but how we respond to them dictates our future karma, whether good or bad. So the practice of yoga by developing stability, calm and clarity, helps us to respond skilfully to the karmic circumstances of our life and to generate good karma for the future. Not only can we transform our bad karma into good karma, we can even free ourselves from karma altogether. This is in fact one of the goals of yoga: to liberate us from the karmic bonds that bind us to the never-ending cycle of birth and death to which we are all subject.

The essence of karma is that whatever we experience is the result of our past actions. It is the operation of impartial, universal justice. Karma shapes our lives from the moment we are born, and before, for the significance of birth and death in the light of karma are simply that they are doorways – doorways to life, in which we reap the karmic fruit of past action and sow the karmic seeds of future experiences. This life leads inevitably to another, as a previous one did to this.

The cycle of birth and death is known as *samsara*, the wheel of life. Liberation from samsara is known as *nirvana*. Yoga brings us to nirvana by resolving our karmic debts and by helping us to act without creating fresh karma, whether good or bad. Any karma will bind us to the wheel, so to liberate ourselves from samsara and attain nirvana we must put an end to karma, past and future.

It is the psychological component of our actions that generates the most potent karma, be it good or bad. So, to kill a murderer in order to prevent him from killing others would not produce bad karma, but it would produce a karmic debt which would have to be paid in the future. To offer someone a helping hand while at the same time resenting them and their need for your help produces bad karma on the basis of your resentment, and good karma on the basis of the action. The bad karma will most likely be strongest, for it is quite likely that the resentment preceded and continued beyond the action itself.

To become free from karma we must learn to act without reacting; we must learn to act with no thought of personal gain, with no trace of personal preference. This is the heart of Karma Yoga, in which all actions are selflessly devoted to God. But karma-free action also arises when we are able to act totally in a given situation without recourse to our habitual processes of analysis, grasping and resisting; when we act with clarity and dispassion with no trace of personal involvement.

This quality of action is learned in meditation practice but is prepared for in asana (yoga postures) and pranayama (breathing). When we sit and allow impressions to arise without reacting with attachment or resistance, without analysis or elaboration, we learn to act from the empty centre of our being. Whenever we are able to attend to a sensation in meditation, or to a situation in life, with our full, undivided and open attention, then we are freeing ourselves from past and future karma. If this becomes our natural and continual way of being then we are free of all karma, we are no longer on the wheel of samsara. We have entered nirvana.

The paradox is, however, that we are still here – we still exist – we still act. For nirvana is not another place; it is not a heaven to which we go when we have established enough merit. The world of nirvana is the world of our everyday life of birth, ageing and death. For those whose actions are determined by karma it is samsara, an endless round of ignorance, fear, greed and hatred that generates suffering. For those who, by cultivating undivided attention in the living of their lives, have released themselves from karmic servitude, it is nirvana, a world of grace and beauty. For those who meet life with only a part of themselves, with divided attention, is it samsara. For those who meet life wholly, with complete attention, it is nirvana. The difference between samsara and nirvana is not one of location but one of awareness. If we are asleep we are bound to the endless wheel of life and death; if we are awake we are free from it.

The wheel of life and death is not only understood as the cycle of death and rebirth, it also has a psychological counterpart. When we are asleep to the conditioned nature of our motivations and attachments, we are locked into a self-perpetuating cycle of attachment and aversion. This cycle is made up of unconscious patterns of thought, desire and action to which we are bound. We continually repeat patterns of thought and behaviour that bind us to a narrow, repetitive life, and mask us from our true potential.

THE ILLUSION OF MAYA

Many people think that yoga is a withdrawal from the world in which a detachment is cultivated which leads to isolation. Although this may be the effect of faulty practice it is not the intention of yoga. Yoga means union, not separation. The underlying psychology of yoga is sophisticated but simple. A key concept is illusion, or *maya*. Maya is a sanskrit term which refers to the unreal world in which we life. Many have taken this to mean that the world in which we live – of material bodies, birth and death – is not real.

In fact maya refers to the tendency of our minds to develop and hold on to conceptual images. These images result from past experience held in our memories. Every experience tends to be stored as a tapestry of images which feed off and into those remaining from other experiences. Long before childhood is over we have built up a complex, sophisticated web of images in our mind. This web is so powerful that we begin to impose it between ourselves and our experiences. When we do this we are no longer experiencing reality. Instead we are projecting an image, based on our past experience, and are living in a world of abstract images rather than concrete reality. This is the illusion of maya.

For example, we may have had an early experience of being attacked by a dog that was painful and frightening. The fear and pain may create such a strong impression on the mind in association with the image of dogs that we become frightened whenever we see a dog, even when there is no danger or aggression in that particular dog. We have created an unconscious image or concept of dogs as dangerous, and this image is so powerful that we are not able to be open to any new experience of a dog. Instead we have to impose between a new dog and ourselves our old image. This is illusion.

This crystalizing tendency of the mind, by which the free and fluid energy of life is frozen into conceptual images which we use as buffers against the unpredictability of the world, dominates most of us most of the time. As we grow older, the weight of images resulting from past experience increases and this weight generates more and more force, until eventually the pressure of accumulated images becomes more powerful than the appeal of objective reality. As adults we rarely have the spontaneous wonder that was our natural state as a child. We are less curious, less adventurous, less expressive. We have become burdened with memories that restrict us.

'THAT THOU ART' – ATMAN AND BRAHMAN

Underlying the conceptual framework with which we buffer the world is a central illusion. This is the illusion of the separate self: of our independent existence. One of the reasons we cling to the crystallized images of the world is that they reinforce our sense of ourself; when the other is clearly defined, so is the self. This is the illusion, that we exist in isolated separateness from everything else, that leads to desire, attachment, and suffering. That there is no absolute and separate individual self does not mean there can therefore be no suffering. This is another illusion that many cling to. If there is no self, they say, there is no-one to experience suffering, so there is no problem to be overcome, no changes to be made, all is a dream. This attitude becomes an excuse for complacent self-indulgence, and could not be further from the spirit of yoga. Suffering is a reality that comes about not by a quirk of fate or external forces beyond our control, but from the attitudes and beliefs that we carry with us unnecessarily.

However, the point is that the illusion is not of pain, suffering or existence, but of a separate, permanent self. What yoga teaches is that there is no self separate from the experience, there is no self-existent subject. There is no subject and no object. There is just being, just existence. The existence of laughter, of tears, of a tree falling, a mountain piercing the clouds. Yoga allows us to cut through the frozen web of images that suggests a separation of subject and object, of self and other, and access the experience of life directly. We learn to live without the filter of the mind's projections, in and as the electrifying energy of each moment. When we do not separate ourselves from the moment as if we were some self-sustaining, self-defined observer, we enter into the ecstasy and harmony of life. As we begin to taste that ecstasy and harmony the power of our illusions, the sense of our separate clinging self, melts away.

Then, rather than being separate from the world, we become one with it. Just as this state of union is the goal and fruit of yoga, so it is its method. We learn to become one with our experience: to dispense with the filtering mechanism which we use as a protection against pain and the unknown. In the practice of asana, we become one with each part of our body. In the experience of meditation, we become one with every state of mind that arises. We do not fight against ourselves, we do not resist the reality of our body and mind, we accept and embrace what we find. To become one with all that we contain is to realize *Atman*, our hidden, true nature. So too must we become one with the world. We do not resist or fight but embrace it. Done with awareness of the tendencies of our mind this can lead to freedom; done blindly and impulsively it leads to further bondage. Atman is often translated as the higher self. However, this is a linguistic contradiction. The very word 'self' depends upon the existence of some external entity opposite to the self: the other. However, the experience of Atman reveals this to be nothing more than a trick of the conditioned mind. The experience of Atman, or 'self', is also the experience of the world as spiritual energy, of *Brahman* – Brahman being the immanent source and foundation of all existence and of which all physical and spiritual manifestations are a fleeting expression. To become one is to become the one next to which there is no other. This is sometimes referred to as 'Tat Tvam Asi' which means 'That Thou Art'.

DESIRE AND ATTACHMENT

The cords that bind us to our deluded sense of our separate self are attachment and desire. Because this is so, many try to give up desire and attachment through denial. This is usually fruitless, however, for the power of desire and attachment comes from our sense of ourself as separate and, to the extent that we live from that illusion, we will continue to have attachment and desire. Therefore, to deny desire is only to repress the energy that arises from our sense of self. When this energy is repressed from our consciousness it lurks in our subconscious, where it releases itself through unconscious thoughts, dreams and actions. In this state the energy of desire can be even more potent and dangerous than when it is conscious. Restricted, it becomes intensified and can produce patterns of behaviour that are in conflict with our conscious intentions. For example, repressed anger can produce a critical tendency in the mind that is dismissive of others so inherently that it goes unnoticed. Repressed fear can diminish our natural curiosity and our willingness to interact with others, leading to isolation.

Instead of repressing desire and denying attachment we have to work with them. The energy they contain can be transformed without having to indulge or repress desires. This transformation comes about when we are able to cultivate spaciousness in our mind that allows us to see the mechanism of desire and attachment. By turning our attention inwardly, we notice the patterns of motivation and assumption from which desires arise. As we see deeper into these patterns they begin to lose their intensity. The energy that is usually concentrated in the impulse of a random desire becomes extended, through our awareness, into the complex pattern of relationships that surrounds that desire. As our awareness takes in the context, the implications, the source of that desire, its intensity diminishes and effortlessly we let go. Then there is neither denial nor indulgence. The energy of desire becomes harnessed to our awareness and generates clarity.

The quality of awareness cultivated in yoga, *samadhi*, is a very special one. As it becomes enriched it reveals certain surprising characteristics. One is rapture, another is peace. These qualities, which result from the accumulation of energy in awareness, or from concentration, soon begin to provide a satisfaction and contentment that chasing after desires never could. Ironically, through the spontaneous restraining action of deeper awareness arises a pleasure greater than any that desire can offer. As this rapture and peace deepen, the energy of desire becomes less and less, and so attachment to both desire and the objects of desire drops away. Then we begin to taste freedom, or *moksha*. The highest state of samadhi is sahaja samadhi, in which the yogin, having been liberated from delusion and realized his true nature, lives freely in the world of samsara without bondage.

Freedom, or moksha, is not a state of isolation or physical detachment. It is one in which we enjoy any situation, event, perception or experience equally through the quality of our awareness. We have learned that by cultivating an unrestricted awareness, by opening widely to experience, we access an energy of pleasure that belongs not to external objects but to the quality of our attention. When the energy of body, breath and mind are completely focused in the task at hand there is a rapture that belongs to us rather than the situation. This is the seventh limb of Ashtanga Yoga, *dhayana*, or absorption. When totally absorbed in our activity, whatever it may be, that is yoga. Then we no longer need to classify experiences and objects into pleasant and unpleasant, we no longer have to desire and reject. Instead we can bring our open quality of awareness into every moment and find in that the peace and rapture that desire promises but fails to deliver.

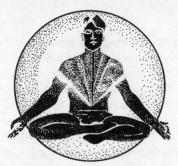

4 . THE FIELD OF ENERGY AND THE SUBTLE BODY

Both the experiential universe of the yogi in exploration of his consciousness and the analysed universe of the quantum physicist's exploration of the nature of matter reveal certain startling properties that seem to conflict with the way in which we habitually perceive reality. What yogis and quantum physicists have discovered is that matter as we know it is a limited phase or function of energy perceived from a particular frame of reference. The frame of reference is that of the externally directed human nervous system. Like all viewpoints it is relative, and colours its perceptions by projecting itself onto its arena of perception. So, while we perceive a tree as solid, if we change our frame of reference and perceive a tree from the point of view of an electron, a neutrino or any of the elusive sub-atomic particles which populate the universe of quantum physicists, it melts into a vortex of dancing, scintillating energy.

One of the observations of both yogis and quantum physicists is that material objects, as fields of energy, do not have the limitation they appear to have when experienced as solid objects held firmly in the three dimensions of space. When we perceive the solid, fixed aspect or nature of an object we tend to see it in isolation from its background, as distinct and separate from everything else. When we see or experience it as a vortex of energy, we no longer make this separation. We realize that the energy of a so-called object is not separate from the energy of its context. While there may appear to be many different, separate objects they are all particular, momentary concentrations of a single vast field of energy. This field of energy, known to yogis as *prakriti, shakti* or the *dance of shiva*, cannot be broken, unravelled or divided. To the limited perception of an undeveloped nervous system intense concentrations of energy appear as solid, separate objects. But this solidity and separateness are only true for a limited viewpoint. Of course, for human beings, as one of those intense concentrations of the universal energy field, it is useful to perceive other objects in this way so that we can operate clearly within the field to which we belong.

For practical purposes it is clearly useful to perceive objects as individual items. However, there are disadvantages as well as advantages in experiencing the indivisible web of energy that makes up the universe as a series of objects in space and events in time. One of these is that we can separate ourselves from the energy of the universe, the energy of life, in our experience. We develop a sense of isolation, separateness, insecurity that inevitably breeds anxiety. This in turn generates the grasping quality of desire that binds us to our sense of self as something separate and to objects as things from which we can squeeze some relief from our insecurity. When we live from this frame of reference, we miss out on the rapturous joy, the ecstasy that is the intrinsic vibration of the universal energy field of which we are a fleeting focus. Just as we are a momentary focus of the energy of the entire universe, so is everything else. What this means is that the power, the delight and the bliss of universal energy is focused, and therefore available, in all objects, all situations. This is true no matter how they may appear to our conditioned minds. When we develop the open, unprejudiced awareness of dhayana this blissful energy becomes our natural experience. Instead of experiencing life as a sequence of events involving separate objects that we like or dislike, we experience life as a dance of energy in which our movements, and those of our partner – the universe, bring wave after wave of ecstasy.

The veil of maya, in which our conceptualization separates self and other, inner and outer, is thick. Its mists keep our thoughts involved in fear and hope, memory and fantasy, obscuring the present. By directing our attention to the concrete actions of the present – the line of the body, the rhythm of the breath, the flow of unrestricted consciousness – yoga begins to dissolve this mist. Then we enter the present, and through the cultivation of inner awareness our lives become our own.

By cultivating inner awareness, or dhayana, we transform our habitual state of consciousness – characterized by anxiety and grasping – into a more profound state in which contentment and detachment, rapture and peace are the stepping stones that lead to the various levels of samadhi. While cultivation of inner awareness begins in the practice of yama, niyama, asana, pranayama and pratyahara, which are the first five limbs of yoga (see chapter 5), it is in meditation that it flowers.

The cultivation of inner awareness is not so much a statement of preference as of making balance. Even when we indulge our imaginations, what we explore is based on external memories and projections. Through yoga we learn to cultivate an inner awareness, not in order to escape from the external world but to embrace it. Our externally directed awareness is usually one of projection, fantasy. We do not directly experience the energy of the world, we impose a shield of maya, of projection. Through cultivating inner awareness we discover genuine outer awareness. By looking inwardly we begin to recognize, and eventually to discard, that deeply ingrained habit of projection which we use as a buffer against direct perception of reality, of the world. So as we cultivate inner awareness, we begin to discover outer awareness. As we look in at the patterns of our mind, we begin to discover the tapestry of life. We find that the movement inwards that we cultivate in yoga is in fact also a movement outwards. We learn to cut through the veil of crystalized conceptualization that masks the world. We discover that the inner and outer world are not separate, unless we artificially separate them with the habitual clamour of our minds.

THE SUBTLE OR ENERGY BODY

We are not made up of only mind and matter, there is also energy. Yoga reveals that we have a subtle energetic counterpart to our physical body which is known as the subtle or energy body. In fact we have five sheaths, or *koshas*: anatomical, energetic, mental, intuitive and blissful. The anatomical body, derived from food, is known as the gross body or physical sheath. The blissful sheath is known as the causal body and is our innermost sheath; this body is the energy of ecstasy that vibrates within us without pause. When we are in conscious contact with it through yoga it illuminates and uplifts us. In between is the subtle body, made up of the energetic, mental and intuitive sheaths. Yoga seeks to release us from attachment to and identification with any and all of these sheaths, so that we can be liberated into the free and unrestricted reality of our true nature, Atman/Brahman.

Matter and energy are like the head and tail of a coin. In Tantra, Kundalini and Hatha Yoga this becomes very significant. Many of their techniques use the physical body to activate the complementary energy systems. Knowledge of the subtle human energy system is not theoretical or speculative, philosophical or allegorical. It is empirical and pragmatic: emerging from direct experience. Direct experience of the energy body is not, however, easy to come by. It requires an awakening of subsensory perception. This perceptual awakening occurs as a matter of course through the correct practice of yoga techniques.

The energy system is composed of *prana*, flowing in channels called *nadis*, controlled and distributed by energy centres known as *chakras*. Prana is the underlying vital energy of the universe. It has many phases or aspects, in much the same way as matter can be differentiated into a wide range of elements. One aspect of prana underlies the physical properties of matter itself, creating and sustaining its structures. In another aspect of it is the life force itself which, in the case of animals and vegetables, animates and vitalizes certain physical structures which we call organisms. In another it takes the form of sentience or consciousness. These can be called structural prana, vital prana, and sentient prana. Without structural prana there can be no stability to permit physical matter to create structures. Without vital prana there cannot be the adaptability and flexibility to permit physical structures to grow, change and decay. Without sentient prana there cannot be the sensitivity to permit organic matter to perceive, to feel, to know.

Inside the physical body prana has five major functions, each regulated by a different aspect: assimilation controlled by *prana*; elimination by *apana*; circulation by *vyana*; expression by *udana*; digestion by *samana*. These are the five inner winds, of which prana and apana are the most important for well being. They must be balanced. If prana predominates there is an excess of energy which can create stress, hyperactivity and tension. If apana predominates there is lassitude, tiredness and a lack of vitality. They are regulated and balanced through asana (yoga posture) and pranayama (breathing). The five winds are also related intimately to the mind, so that their motion is reflected in the movement of the mind. By balancing prana and apana through pranayama, the mind becomes quiet and ready for meditative absorption.

There are yoga techniques for accumulating, generating, stabilizing and directing prana of each kind. These techniques are not only the means to create a potent energy body but also to nourish our physical body and stabilize our consciousness. By creating a more stable and potent energy body the yogi seeks to transcend the inherent limitations of his physical body. He can then learn to use the physical body in ways beyond the norm by transforming it through his energy body. While many esoteric instances of this are known, they also include more simple things such as healing disease, slowing down the heart and the blood, and changing local body temperatures.

The three main nadis through which prana flows are called

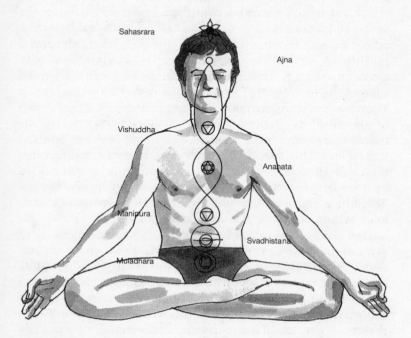

The subtle body showing chakras and nadis

ida, pingala and *sushumna*, otherwise known respectively as the currents of Moon, Sun and Fire, and are located in the region of the spinal column. Sushumna lies to the centre and ida and pingala curl around it from the bottom to the top, crossing the spine and meeting each other at six of the seven major chakras. One of the effects and aims of Hatha, Tantra and Kundalini Yoga is to balance the charge of prana in ida and pingala until an awakening of sushumna occurs, which is experienced as the raising of the serpent power dormant at the root of the spine, kundalini. This awakening is a powerful and dramatic experience that occurs only after sincere and dedicated practice. It brings about a radical transformation of mind and body that is marked and clearly observable.

Related to ida, pingala, sushumna and kundalini are the seven major chakras. In the pelvic floor is Muladhara Chakra, where lies dormant the coiled kundalini. Svadhistana Chakra is a little higher. In the region of the navel is Manipura Chakra. In the heart region is Anahata Chakra. In the throat is Vishuddha Chakra. In between the eyebrows is Ajna Chakra, which is known as the third eye and is the seat of wisdom. In the crown of the head is Brahma Chakra or Sahasrara Chakra, the thousand-petalled lotus. The chakras are nourished, cleansed and balanced by the practice of asana and pranayama. Through the application of the bandhas and mudras, kundalini is guided up through the chakras until it awakens the crown chakra. This brings about the deepest awakening of human consciousness, which is cosmic consciousness.

The human imagination is potent and vivid and human aspirations are often intense. Consequently, many yoga students delude themselves into imagining that they can feel nadis and chakras and have awakened kundalini, when in fact they are simply beginning to tune in to subtle vibrations of the central nervous system that are usually imperceptible. Nevertheless, it *is* possible to experience the subtle energy body when the anatomical body is stable, the mind is quiet, and attention is focused deeply and openly.

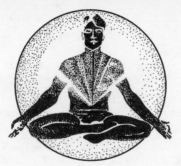

5 · THE LIMBS OF ASHTANGA YOGA: 1–5

FIRST LIMB OF YOGA: YAMA

Yama is the observance of psychological restraint. It is the first limb of yoga because all our actions are coloured by our underlying motivations. Yama comprises five restraining tendencies, which are not absolute moral commandments but psychological buttresses to a still mind, without which progress in yoga will elude us.

Those who attempt to perfect the practice of yama without the internalizing practice of asana, pranayama and dharana (see below) will be hard pressed, for the practice of yama alone is often a struggle against our conditioning. But consistent practice of the inner limbs of yoga will lead effortlessly to the manifestation of yama.

Yama makes us conscious of the powerful and automatic nature of our desires. The so-called morality of yama is the natural expression of self-knowledge in which the compulsive nature of desire and attachment, and the anxiety they generate, become transparent to the extent that they no longer exert such influence on our behaviour. Once we are conscious of the destructive tyranny of desire we soon let go of it simply by becoming aware of it as the hot brick that it is.

NON-VIOLENCE

Non-violence is more than restraining from physical force. Violent thoughts, such as those of anger or resentment, also disturb the mind. Equally damaging is gossip. Both verbalized gossip and inner gossip are destructive to equanimity of mind.

HONESTY

While honesty means to refrain from telling lies it also means not hiding the truth from others and ourselves. So much of our thought is taken up with distortion of our feelings and intentions in order to be acceptable or in order not to be exposed. It is a part of the practice of honesty to examine our actions, our words and our thoughts, and refrain from any distortion of the truth.

NON-STEALING

Non-stealing also means not taking that which is not freely given. Through it patience and humility are also cultivated.

CONTINENCE

Rather than implying celibacy, this restraint refers to not indulging in sex as a means of escaping from awareness. So much sexual activity, whether physical or in fantasy, is pursued solely as a means to escape from the boredom or discomfort of reality.

NON-COVETING

The satisfaction of desire by external objects or situations is always temporary. It is soon followed by discontent which leads to more and more desire. Only by letting go of desire for what we do not have can the mind become quiet and allow the cultivation of inner awareness that leads to the goal of yoga.

SECOND LIMB OF YOGA: NIYAMA

Niyama, the second limb of yoga, comprises the five qualities needed as a basis for yoga practice. These qualities provide the driving fuel that ignites and drives the yogi on his way. Without them the rigours of practice become daunting, doubt creeps in, and practice becomes intermittent and insincere until it is dropped altogether.

PURITY

Purity of body, mind and action are essential to yoga. The body, nourished by health-giving foods, must be a source of strength and energy. Purity of mind is brought about through the practice of yama. Purity of action is when the mind and body are fully engaged on the task in hand; there is no separation between mental and physical activity. Along with the physical purity that brings good health and the psychological purity cultivated through the practice of yama, purity of action is vital to yoga practice. It is of little value to practise yogic techniques absent-mindedly, or while wishing to be in another time or place.

CONTENTMENT

The ability to be content with little is vital to yoga practice. A mind that is driven by desire for more will be unable to stay still enough or present enough to enter deeply into the practice of yoga. If we have no contentment we are unable to motivate ourselves to establish the stillness and quietness basic to yoga practice. If we are able to practise yoga, then contentment naturally follows from our regular practice as it erodes the binding of desire, and releases us from the habitual anxiety that desire generates.

COMMITMENT

The yogi must have commitment to his practice; if not he will be inconsistent and will never benefit from the fruit of his efforts. The pressures and distractions of life are so constant and so potent that their effects cannot be avoided other than by constant redirection of our awareness into the present. If we stop our practice then we soon slip back into the thrall of desire and attachment and its false promise of happiness.

SELF-KNOWLEDGE

As the yogi progresses self-knowledge automatically develops. This knowledge, both of limitations and limitlessness, problems and potentials, aids in practice and helps to maintain the necessary commitment.

SURRENDER

In the beginning the yogi must surrender to the methods of yoga. With regular practice this surrender becomes more and more natural as we let go of the grasping quality of mind that kept us bound to desire. When our surrender is complete, when we are no longer concerned with establishing external security and happiness, the inner security that yoga offers arises.

THE THIRD LIMB OF YOGA: ASANA

Asana, the third limb of yoga, is a term describing the series of physical postures which are an integral part of the practice of yoga. However, there is a subtle but profound difference between yoga asana and a stretch exercise: the former is characterized by a combination of physical alignment and mental awareness, whereas the latter is merely a gymnastic exercise. By establishing the correct alignment of each part of the body, only achieved by directing the attention inwardly throughout the whole body, posture becomes asana. (See pp. 78–103, where the asana postures are described and illustrated.)

We all carry individual patterns of tension in the muscles. The uneven action of the muscles on the skeleton pulls at bones and joints, displacing them. This in turn intensifies the muscular imbalance and tension by forcing some muscles to work harder than others to compensate. These patterns of imbalance become deeply entrenched, to the extent that if they are disturbed it can feel awkward to us. Our sense of our physical self is moulded around our own patterns of postural imbalance. If we simply try to get the greatest possible extension in a stretch, we may become more flexible but we may also further entrench our postural imbalances. The hidden tensions that these imbalances create, so much a part of us that we do not notice them, remain. We can also overstretch muscles to the point of straining them.

In asana, by developing an awareness of the alignment of the whole body we ensure that stretches are not only balanced but also that, in holding the posture, we release patterns of postural imbalance. This ensures that each body part carries its own share of the action in a posture without any areas of overload or stress.

Aligning the body correctly, which requires a considerable effort of attention, has a powerful mental effect, as it only comes through awareness of each part of the body simultaneously. It awakens the somatic intelligence, uniting mind and body. When awareness is fully in the action, then the action is complete, balanced and effortless.

This harmonizing of mind and body is the beginning of the fruit of yoga, the opening of the spiritual doorway. When mind and body overcome their functional duality and operate in unison, tremendous energy is released and made available. Conversely when yoga is practised mechanically or absent-mindedly, besides the risk of injury there is a loss of energy: the postures can be exhausting. For if parts of the body are unconscious, dull or inactive, then other parts must overwork to compensate which creates tension and a loss of available energy.

Through alignment and awareness posture becomes asana, stretch becomes yoga. To liberate the mind it must be released from its patterns of hidden tension which are reflected in the body. So the practice of yoga must begin on a physical level. The universal awareness of higher consciousness can only ripen if the roots of physical and mental harmony are cultivated. This can only be done by establishing correct alignment and awakening the intelligence throughout the whole body.

THE FOURTH LIMB OF YOGA: PRANAYAMA

Pranayama is more than simply breathing exercises, for it involves activating, harmonizing and intensifying the hidden energy of the life-force, known as *prana*. Without prana there is no life. Prana is the vehicle of consciousness and the energy of matter. The purpose of pranayama practice is to master the movement of prana within us. (See pp. 103–8 for description of how to practice pranayama.)

While we take in prana all the time through food and air, we are also constantly losing it in physical action, mental effort, emotional activity. If output is greater than input, then we become tired and eventually prone to disease. The basic purpose of pranayama is to ensure an adequate intake of prana through the respiratory system. Pranayama allows us to assimilate more of the prana from the air that we breathe and thereby increases our physical and mental energy. Our lungs and nervous system must be resilient and stable enough to hold the increased current of prana; if they are not, then excess prana becomes dangerous and can lead to physical and mental imbalances.

The physiological purpose of pranayama is to improve the oxygenation, purification and circulation of blood and lymph. Respiration has two aspects. The outer aspect is exchanging gases between our blood and the air in the lungs; the inner aspect is exchanging gases between our blood and every cell in our body. When we inhale to the lungs, the cells expire carbon dioxide into the venous blood. When we exhale from our lungs, our cells are inhaling oxygen from our blood. In order to purify every cell of waste products and to provide it with adequate oxygen, we must use our lungs fully. The more deeply we breathe, the more oxygen is available. This vitalizes every cell in our body and our vital organs, nervous system and specialized cells become more efficient. We become healthier.

By bringing to the cells the oxygen that they need to assimilate nutrients pranayama develops a physical and mental vitality that becomes the root of good health and clear judgement. Deep breathing is a generator of energy. If our breath is shallow and unsteady, we find difficulty in maintaining adequate metabolic energy to ensure our health. Then the energy that we use for physical and mental activities drains our vitality and our vital organs and bodies become weak. If however, we ensure a metabolic surplus of energy, we will have abundant reserves of energy for mental, creative, social and professional activities. This we can only do by ensuring both an adequate supply of nutrients through a sensible, natural diet and by regular, deep breathing. By spending some time daily practising to extend the capacity of our lungs, our normal, habitual breathing becomes deeper and more consistent.

One aspect of the breath that is so fundamental that we take it for granted is its relationship to our emotions. When we are upset or anxious, our breath becomes disturbed: it may be suspended, short and sharp, or heavy and laboured. We can calm disturbed emotions simply by regulating our breath. Just taking a deep breath and letting it out slowly relaxes the body and mind by activating the relaxation response of the parasympathetic nervous system. Pranayama therefore tends to generate a more tranquil, calm state of mind in which we are less prone to extreme or unpredictable emotional responses. By learning to control the flow of breath we are also learning to harmonize, calm and quieten the mind.

THE FIFTH LIMB OF YOGA: PRATYAHARA

Although there are at least two exercises specific to the practice of pratyahara, sanmukhi mudra (see p. 59) and savasana (see p. 66), it is mainly developed through the correct practice of asana and pranayama. Pratyahara means internalization of awareness by withdrawal of the senses from contact with the world. This is a prerequisite to accomplishment in both asana and pranayama. Through them it is cultivated, and the ability to maintain clear consciousness with the nervous system directed internally is developed to a point where the practice of effective meditation becomes possible. When the yogi has developed skill in pratyahara, the subtle rigour of meditation becomes much easier. Those who have not developed pratyahara, through the cultivation of inner awareness in asana and pranayama, find the advanced yoga techniques of meditation much more difficult and less fruitful, for a mind not prepared may find meditation frustrating, boring and discouraging. While these states of mind are not in themselves hindrances to meditation many people find it difficult to accept them. Having initially cultivated stability in asana, and tranquillity in pranayama these states are more easily accepted.

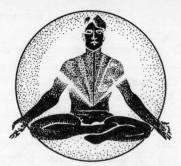

6 · THE LIMBS OF ASHTANGA YOGA: 6–8

Meditation is the heart of yoga. Of the eight limbs of yoga, the last three are specifically concerned with meditation. Through concentration (dharana), we arrive at a state of absorption (dhayana); when this is sustained, we are released from our limited sense of our self and transcend our habitual dualistic state of consciousness (samadhi).

One of the great misconceptions regarding meditation is that to meditate we must stop all thought. Another is that to meditate is to create a state of altered consciousness in which peace and joy predominate, which is really a description of the *result* of meditation – the final stage of yoga – samadhi. To meditate as a deliberate, conscious act is not to stop all thought and create a subtle mind state. The essence of meditation, as of all the limbs of yoga, is union, not separation. So, when we sit to meditate we do not set up an artificial separation between our self-awareness and our thoughts. Nor do we deny or reject whatever emotions or mental states we may find when we begin to closely observe the content of our minds.

The actual experience of meditation is to cultivate a profound, living awareness of the mechanism of our mind. Thereby we begin to lose our attachment to habitual thought patterns, mind states, emotions and ideas, which we cling to as a means of identifying ourselves in external noises. We simply observe the pattern and tendency of our mind. We notice our response to external stimuli. But we do so openly, generously, without evaluation, judgement or analysis. We just observe and allow. In effect the process of meditation is one in which we make friends with ourselves in a very deep way. This we do by refraining from any tendency to criticize, judge, deny or repress the activity of our minds.

However, this is not to say that we just sit passively watching our minds go by. There is a balance between spontaneity (the natural activity of the mind no longer being analysed and classified), and discipline (concentrating the attention to bring the mind into the simple activity of the present). Just as asana and pranayama began the process of unifying mind and body, so meditation deepens and refines this process. Through meditation we first accept the surface levels of our mind then — with practice, as our ability to focus our minds develops — we begin to penetrate deeper levels of our consciousness. As we do this we begin to uncover the qualities of rapture, peace and compassion that are the natural characteristics of our mind. These qualities become lost to us as we become locked into crystalized patterns of grasping and aversion. Observing the subtle mechanisms that keep our minds in a state of externally directed anxiety, we let go of them and get in touch with the deeper, nurturing qualities of mind that lay hidden beneath.

Meditation is more than a technique for creating a special mind state. It is a process in which all of our mind states are revealed. Peace and bliss may well be the natural expression of our uncluttered minds, but they are not habitual. Before these deeper aspects of our consciousness emerge we must acknowledge and assimilate all the more superficial aspects. So the process of making friends with ourselves is one in which we more often than not initially experience uncomfortable mind states: boredom, pain, fear, loneliness, guilt, anger. When we have integrated these experiences and mind states without prejudice, without judgement, then a quietness begins to develop in our minds that allows the deeper, more nourishing mind qualities to emerge. While it is possible to force special mind states – whether through drugs, hypnosis or special exercises – this is not yoga; it does not promote freedom but a dependency on the technique.

THE SIXTH LIMB OF YOGA: DHARANA

Dharana is the first phase of meditation. The more it has been cultivated in asana, pranayama and pratyahara the more productive will be the practice of meditation. The many techniques for the practice of dharana all embody one principle: this is the use of a 'seed' to narrow the activity of the mind to a single point (see pp. 110–12). In effect there are two kinds of seed: those that can be directly perceived (sensation-based seeds) and those that need to be imagined. Because the former are a natural part of our experience, and require no invention, they are generally more fruitful. The purpose of yoga is not to invent something but to discover the way things actually are in their deepest, fullest, most subtle aspects.

The simplest and most common seed is the action and effect of the breath. When focusing on the breath, it should be experienced from the lower abdomen. Not only is this the seat of our breath, it is also our physical centre. This area of the lower abdomen is also understood to be the location of reserves of prana or life-force, the seat of our vitality. So, by sitting with a strong, stable posture that is grounded in this area and by focusing our attention into it we unite our physical, energy and mental bodies in our awareness of their mutual centre. By focusing our awareness on the movement of our breath in our lower abdomen we instantly unite body, mind and breath.

It is important to find a balance in our practice of dharana. The mind should be like a bowstring strung on a piece of willow. It should have tone, without being tight or loose. If too tight it will create tension; if too loose it will wander. The seed of breath is not a focus that we must maintain at all costs; rather it is a frame on which we weave the energy of our mind into patterns of concentration and absorption. It is therefore unhelpful to fight the natural arising of thoughts and feelings, as it is to perceive external stimuli as disturbances. We should accept all movements of our mind, originating inside or outside, without prejudice. We use the need not as a means to deflect inner and outer experience but as a means to concentrate our minds so as to better enter into the richness of each moment.

Dharana is a technique for exercising and developing the mind. It allows us to focus our attention and develop deep concentration. Having made an agreement to follow our seed, when we notice that our mind has wandered it will automatically come back. As our practice deepens we begin earlier to notice our minds wandering. Soon we can notice a single thought arising and return to our seed before developing it into a loquacious ramble that we do not intend. Eventually we begin to notice the impulse that generates a thought, and in noticing it we return to our seed with our attention concentrated more deeply through having absorbed the energy that would have ripened into a thought process. It is especially at this point that dharana begins to become dhayana, and the fruit of practice begins to ripen.

THE SEVENTH LIMB OF YOGA: DHAYANA

Dhayana is not initially a technique that can be practised; it is a consequence of dharana. When we are able to remain focused on our seed, the energy of our body is united with the energies of our mind. This union of the considerable energy of mind and body cuts through the habitual frantic activity of mind and reveals a quality of awareness that in its stillness embraces deep peace and vibrant joy. At this level the object of meditation acts as a focus for the mind, in which the energies of mind are united and reveal their innate qualities. In our daily life any situation or object can act in the same way, absorbing our attention fully and bringing us into a state of dhayana.

Dhayana occurs when the energy generated by dharana flowers through the focus of the seed and connects to the energy of the entire universe of which the seed is a transient focus. In everyday life this quality of awareness, in which attention is gathered and penetrating but narrow, is more likely to occur when we are inactive than when we are active – perhaps when we are relaxing quietly with no intent, or waiting in a queue, or involved in some automatic activity such as driving. Sometimes, provided our practice has generated enough concentration of energy and established a deep enough level of stillness, our awareness spontaneously flowers into dhayana. Sometimes this flowering is momentary; sometimes it can last days or weeks, perhaps only being noticeable in the pauses between our activities when our mind is free from discriminating focus. It is usually characterized by tranquillity, rapture, vitality and contentment.

When dhayana has arisen spontaneously, and our concentration is sufficiently strong, it is possible to generate it at will. We are able to move from dharana quickly into dhayana. The transition from fragmented consciousness to deep absorption can be made deliberately. However, this requires considerable preparation and is rarely possible without great dedication to practice.

THE EIGHTH LIMB OF YOGA: SAMADHI

When dhayana deepens, the sense of oneself as separate from the seed falls away. In samadhi the seed reveals the true nature of both itself and our awareness as being foci of the energy of the whole universe. In this revelation subject and object disappear and the ecstatic energy of the universe is revealed unhindered by limited perceptions. The freedom of samadhi is not one of escape, it is one of experiencing reality directly without the filters of the mind's projections, without preference or judgement.

Samadhi is a state of being which can only be understood through experience. Any description can be no more than a finger pointing at the moon. This is because the full implications of reality, of freedom, of enlightenment cannot be grasped by the dualistic mind. The mind and its conceptual demarcations of this and that, self and other, is and is not, is inadequate to embrace the rich contours of reality. This richness often appears to the limited, dualistic mind as contradiction, paradox or confusion. However, it is not reality that is confusing or paradoxical but our descriptions of it.

When we experience life without filter, then we are free, then we are in samadhi. When we project a screen of mental clutter between ourselves and the world, then we are in bondage. As we practise yoga we experience moments of freedom, which will alternate with times of bondage. To cling to freedom, to long for it, even to strive for it is to be in bondage, to be caught up in our mind's projections and missing the abundant beauty of the moment's bounty. We find freedom not in certainty, not in permanence, but in embracing the uncertainty of impermanence. So, we do not practise to gain anything extra, to add the final feather to our caps. We practise simply to be here, to be alive, awake to the moment, whatever it offers us.

SAMYAMA

In the Yoga Sutras Patanjali describes the process of meditation – the continuity between dharana, dhayana and samadhi – as *samyama*. Both Buddhist and yoga texts classify dharana, dhayana and samadhi into various levels of absorption. Dharana is defined as holding the mind still for 12 seconds; dhayana as holding the mind still for 12×12 seconds, or 2.5 minutes; samadhi as holding the mind still for 12×12×12 seconds or 36 minutes. While this is a little technical it gives some idea of the relationship between them. It is important to realize that holding the mind still for even 12 seconds is a formidable achievement and requires diligent practice.

In the traditional classifications of absorption, various mind states are described. One important practical aspect of these graded levels of absorption is that some of them involved thought. It is important to recognize thought as a natural activity of the mind that is being harnessed rather than something to be stopped. Without thought we cannot even begin yoga practice. Because thought does not interfere with absorption it is possible to be in a state of dhayana or samadhi even in daily life. This is an important consideration for those whose pursuit of yoga is not an escape from the world but an exploration of its more subtle aspects.

ADDITIONAL TECHNIQUES

MUDRA, BANDHA AND DRUSHTI

While these are practical techniques for complete yoga practice they require direct assistance from a teacher to be learned properly and safely. Therefore we do not recommend that you try them on your own. They are included here so as to give an overall view of yoga practice. This does not apply to the finger gestures which can safely be practised alone.

BANDHAS

Bandha means a lock or seal. Bandhas are inner techniques vital to the effectiveness and safety of asana and pranayama as they ensure that concentration and prana are not dissipated but maintained within. Their effect is more than physiological, for they have a profound effect on the subtle energy body and the flow of prana. Without their use yoga will never bear its more subtle fruits. There are three major bandhas. They are not only used in the practice of pranayama, where they are essential, but also in the practice of asana and meditation, where they help to unify the physical, energy and mental bodies.

Mula bandha

This is the root lock. It is necessary for penetrating the esoteric aspect of yoga. It involves awakening a small group of nerves in the pelvic floor, which is the anatomical counterpart of the root chakra muladhara. When this has been awakened by mastering the muscles of the pelvic floor, it leads to an awakening of the energy body and the kundalini. Through mula bandha yoga transforms physical, especially sexual, energy into subtle, spiritual energy. Mula bandha also has an important anatomical effect. Contracting the muscles in the pelvic floor creates resistance in the lower back, abdominals, sacro-iliac joints, adductors, hamstrings and quadriceps. This makes it difficult to overstretch and damage these muscles by over-exertion.

Uddiyana bandha

Known as the lion that overcomes the elephant death, uddiyana means flying up. It is used to direct the energy generated in asana and pranayama, especially by the action of mula bandha, upwards. Otherwise this energy remains low down in the body and can lead to over-identification with the physical world in general and sexual energy in particular. On a physiological level it massages, tones and cleanses the abdominal organs making them strong and healthy. It also restores elasticity to the lungs and massages the heart through its hollowing effect on the thorax. It is said to restore youthfulness. It is done by drawing the abdominal wall in and up as far as possible towards the spine, when the lungs are empty. A similar but less intense action, which draws the abdominal wall in and stabilizes it, is known as uddiyana mudra, and can be done throughout all phases of respiration.

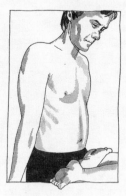 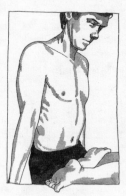 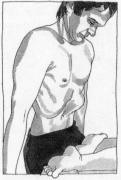

| *Normal* | *Uddiyana* | *Uddiyana* |
| *abdomen* | *mudra* | *bandha* |

Jalandhara bandha

This is the net-holding lock, done by lowering the chin onto the breastbone and contracting the throat. This is vital when holding the breath with lungs full so as to avoid pressure above the glottis. It depends upon the softening and lengthening of the upper back and neck muscles so that it can be done without tension. It also stimulates the three nerves that

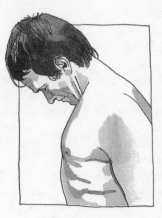

Jalandhara bandha

emerge from the spinal column in the throat that control the diaphragm. Its esoteric purpose is to prevent the downward flow, and loss, of the spiritual ambrosia, *amrita*, which is released by the crown chakra. If it is swallowed it is destroyed by the gastric fire. This ambrosia can be tasted during yoga, especially during extended periods in inverted postures.

All these bandhas are necessary when practising the subtle techniques of pranayama and should be practised from the beginning in order to be able to use them effectively when they are necessary. Mula bandha must be prepared for through the practice of combining aswini and vajroli mudra, outlined below, (see p. 57). Uddiyana can be prepared for with kapalabhati, also defined below, (see p. 61). Jalandhara is prepared for by the shoulderstand sequence (see pp. 97–8).

MUDRAS

The mudras are gestures. These gestures can be very subtle, such as the joining of fingertips, or more comprehensive, such as applying all of the three bandhas together. They are also used to seal or circulate energy in specific areas or channels and bring about an effect on consciousness through the energy body rather than the physical body.

Mahamudra is a combination of mula bandha, uddiyana bandha and jalandhara bandha performed in a sitting posture.

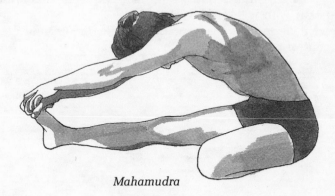

Mahamudra

Uddiyana mudra is used throughout asana and pranayama to stabilize the lungs. It is done by drawing the lower abdominal wall beneath the navel in towards the spine.

Aswini mudra is the alternating contraction and release of the inner and outer anal sphincters, necessary for the mastery of mula bandha. It feels like trying to prevent defecation.

Vajroli mudra is the contraction of the urogenital muscles, also necessary for the mastery of mula bandha. It feels like trying to prevent urination.

Jnana mudra is lightly touching the tip of the index finger to the thumb while sitting for pranayama or samyama. There is a

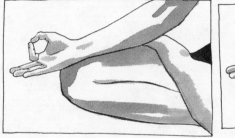
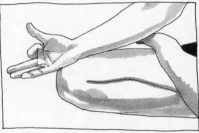

Jnana mudra   *Active jnana mudra*

more active variation of this mudra where the tip of the index finger is pressed into the inside of the knuckle of the thumb.

Vishnu mudra is used in pranayama to manipulate the nostrils. In it the index and middle fingers of the right hand are bent onto the palm, while the other fingers and the thumb control the nostrils.

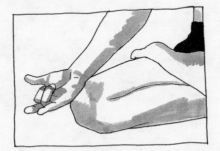

Vishnu mudra

Atmanjali mudra, known as the prayer position, is when the palms are placed together in front of the chest, often used in meditation.

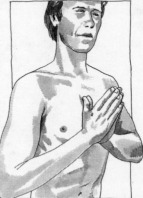

Atmanjali mudra

Dhayana mudra is supporting the left palm in the right just below the navel with the thumb tips lightly joined. This is the main yogic mudra used during Buddhist meditation.

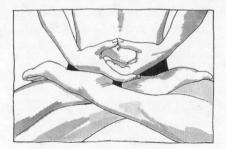

Dhayana mudra

Sanmukhi mudra is used to develop pratyahara. The fingers and thumbs of both hands are used to seal the openings of the face, cutting off external awareness.

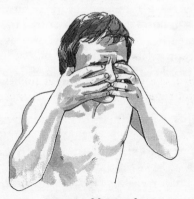

Sanmukhi mudra

DRUSHTI

Like mudras and bandhas, drushti are used to contain energy, but on a more subtle level. A high level of accomplishment and sensitivity is required to feel their effect but at a certain level they are essential. They are gaze points, to which the eyes are directed during asana, pranayama and meditation. Initially these points are external but eventually they are internal. Gazing inwardly at the third eye while meditating is the best-known example. Each asana and pranayama has a specific drushti which helps to contain the energy each one generates. They focus not only the eyes but also the mind.

MANTRA, MANDALA AND YANTRA

Yogis developed a wide range of techniques for focusing the mind to create a meditative state. Two of these are the use of sound in the form of repeated phrases, or mantra, and the use of visual aids to visualization, or yantra.

While the repetition of a sacred mantra may be the whole of one's yoga practice, it is usually a part of a broader sadhana. Mantras can be used to aid asana and pranayama practice as well as meditation. The two most famous mantras are AUM, popular amongst Hindus, and AUM MANI PADME HUM, popular amongst Buddhists.

Aum represents the inner vibration of the cosmos. It has three aspects, each corresponding to one of the Hindu trinity. 'A' represents creation or Brahman, 'U' represents continuity or Vishnu, 'M' represents dissolution or Siva. It is regarded as the most potent and sacred of all mantras. Many other longer mantras begin or end with it.

Mandalas and yantras are more specific to tantric yoga, and in particular Tibetan Buddhism. They involve the creation of geometric shapes and drawings that represent the cosmos in various aspects or in totality. While initially they are used as external visual aids, eventually they are internalized by visualization. This requires highly developed powers of visualization and concentration and is a very advanced practice, not to be confused with vague imaging of New Age creative visualizations. Yantras and mandalas that are internally visualized are extremely complex and are built up rather like a mosaic, or Cezanne painting, point by point until the complete image is supported by the whole of the yogin's consciousness.

SHAT KRIYA

The *shat kriya* are the purification practices used in Hatha Yoga. They cleanse the digestive tract from mucous build-up and keep the internal environment clean and sensitive. However, they are not necessary if the full range of asana are practised as in Ashtanga Vinyasa or Iyengar Yoga in combination with a balanced diet. Many of the yoga asana are designed to stimulate, massage, rinse, drain and cleanse the internal organs of digestion, respiration and elimination.

Three of the shat kriya are quite safe for anyone to practise:

Kapalabahti, meaning shining skull because it cleanses and invigorates the brain, also cleanses the nasal passage, sinuses and lungs. It involves fast forceful abdominal breathing, a little similar to the bhastrika or bellows breath of pranayama. It is not however a pranayama and does not use the complete yoga breath. It is short, shallow and sharp. It is used to waken and cleanse the lungs before pranayama proper. Its practice develops the abdominal muscles, thereby acting as a preparation for nauli and uddiyana.

Nauli involves rolling the abdominal muscles and is very difficult and powerful. It helps in mastering the bandhas, pranayama, vasti and dhauti.

Trataka involves cleansing and developing the eyes with various techniques known as inner, outer and intermediate fixing. The most simple technique is to stare at a candle flame until the eyes water.

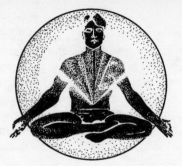

7 · THE EFFECTS OF YOGA

PHYSICAL BENEFITS OF YOGA

Increased suppleness is one of the most immediate benefits of asana practice. The voluntary muscles of the body, which we use for movement, normally have three differing states. They are contraction, when the muscle is working; tone, when the muscle is inactive but not relaxed; relaxed, when the muscle is at rest as in sleep. Asana practice focuses on a fourth less usual state of muscle tone: deep stretch or extension.

In the asana postures every muscle in the body, even those we never normally use, are systematically stretched. While muscles may be stretched in normal activity they are not usually stretched to the maximum, nor held passively. In asana, muscles are given a maximum stretch only achieved by working gradually and slowly. This stretch is then held gently without forcing the muscles. The fibres are able to lengthen naturally and each time they are used in this way they not only lengthen but become more elastic. If muscles are forced this will not happen – the fibres will resist and maximum extension will diminish due to hardening. It is therefore important not to jerk on the muscles while holding the postures.

As the muscles become more flexible they also strengthen

in a unique way. The body itself becomes the gymnasium on which the muscles develop. Each posture uses certain muscles to support, lift or stretch parts of the body against the force of gravity and its own inherent resistance. The body then becomes our set of weights which other parts have to work to lift and support. Rather than pumping the muscles through forced contraction, the muscle fibres are worked in two different ways: one is in stretching, the other is in the controlled and sustained contraction needed to maintain a stretch. This strengthens the muscles not by increasing their bulk but by improving their efficiency. So while yoga develops strength it does not increase bulk. Instead it develops muscular tone that is even and balanced through the whole body.

Many people assume that because yoga is not always a form of moving exercise it does not develop stamina. In fact it requires much more strength and muscular stamina to execute a posture slowly than fast. By holding the postures when they have become more comfortable muscular stamina is developed very quickly. Stamina is especially developed by the standing and inverted postures – the latter often being held for half an hour at a stretch. When postures are connected together into a flowing sequence, as in Ashtanga Vinyasa Yoga, the development of cardiovascular stamina is rapid and impressive.

By working evenly throughout the body – equally on the left and right, the front and back – asana practice realigns every bone in the body. This is achieved by loosening the joints and evenly stretching the muscles, thus releasing residual tension so the bones of the skeleton move freely into their natural position. Hips move into line and vertebrae regain their natural alignment. This naturally improves our posture, promoting a light and graceful bearing. The lightness and openness of our posture is an expression not only of the freedom that we are finding in our body but also in our mind and heart.

The effort required to establish and hold the postures demands deep, smooth, soft breathing. As we work into the postures we find that we need to use the breath by deepening and lengthening it. In doing so we begin to reactivate dormant lung tissue and set up new, more beneficial patterns of breathing. Many of the postures work specifically to open the chest, strengthening the respiratory muscles and loosening and stretching lung tissue. The practice of pranayama further develops lung capacity and retrains both the lungs and the brain to breathe more deeply and effectively. This then improves oxygenation of the blood, which in turn improves cellular metabolism, strengthening and vitalizing every organ in the body.

When stretching, twisting, bending forwards and backwards, various organs are alternately stretched, squeezed or relaxed. In the process they are either rinsed in fresh blood or drained of old blood. This alternate rinsing and draining rejuvenates cellular tissue and improves their vital functioning. Through the rinsing and draining action of asana on the digestive organs their metabolic function is improved and the tone of the muscles of oesophagus, stomach and intestines is maintained. Through improved circulation and respiration cellular vitality is enhanced so that the digestion improves. Some postures exert direct pressure on the large intestine and kidneys, helping the elimination of waste products.

Blood and lymph circulation are also improved by stretching the muscles and by inverted postures. Venous blood flow is produced by muscular activity. By working every muscle in the body asana promotes healthy blood circulation. This ensures adequate cellular metabolism throughout the whole body. Improved respiration also enhances blood circulation as the action of the lungs also supports the heart in pumping blood around the body.

Improved circulation, muscular extension and relaxation nourish the nervous system. The cells of the nervous system are toned and their pathways polished so that their activity is enhanced. The central nervous system in the spinal column benefits especially from the different stretches and movements of the spine, as does the vagus nerve in the front of the body. The various nerve plexi are activated and rinsed in fresh blood. Overall the nervous system not only becomes more vital but also more sensitive. As a result, control over bodily movement becomes more and more refined and subtle. At the same time sensitivity to the subtle actions of the body is developed allowing for even further refinement of control and movement.

Overall, then, yoga practice promotes good health. Every cell of every organ and muscle is invigorated and supplied with fresh blood while being drained efficiently of waste products. There is much less possibility of toxic build-up, either on the cellular level or in the organs themselves. By promoting the health of the organs, including the glands of the immune system, the body's ability to resist disease is enhanced. Body weight is also kept to an optimal level as waste products are discharged, nutrients are fully absorbed and muscle tone is improved. Likewise the skin quality improves as blood circulation is enhanced, bringing a smooth, clear complexion and bright, sparkling eyes.

PSYCHOLOGICAL BENEFITS OF YOGA

Working with the limitations of our mind and body is difficult. The resistance to yoga postures and even to sitting still can be considerable. Through persevering we learn the joy of overcoming obstacles and not giving in to difficulty. This develops an attitude we carry over into our daily lives. So, when confronted with difficulties or hardship we have the resilience to continue without giving up. With this new-found strength, we begin to appreciate ourselves more, to improve our self-esteem. This in turn gives us the confidence to be more ambitious, more engaged with life.

Yoga demands concentration. The process of mastering the postures itself strengthens our concentration and this newly developed power then becomes available to us in daily life. The ability to maintain concentration on a given activity is one of the greatest assets in life. The effect of keeping the mind intently concentrated for extended periods in yoga unifies the often divergent energies of the mind. As our mental energy becomes more unified, various mental faculties, such as memory and recall, begin to improve. This occurs also because yoga releases psychological blocks that impede the mind. When the mind is habitually relaxed, still and unified it tends to function more effectively.

Yoga brings deep relaxation. Because the postures work deeply into muscular tissue, entrenched habitual tension is released. We become aware of the patterns of tension in our body and learn to let go of them consciously in our daily life. This is deepened through pranayama as we begin to let go of emotional tensions locked into thoracic muscles. The practice of savasana (see pp. 98–100) teaches us how to systematically and deeply release tension in every muscle in our body while simultaneously relaxing the mind.

As muscular and emotional tension are released we become calmer and our ability to face life's trials and tribulations is enhanced. We face the world with less anxiety and apprehension. This allows us to perceive, respond and act effectively without being disturbed by emotional over-reactions. We can enjoy the passing moments of our life more fully.

As we begin to relax we become less compulsively attached. So often our attachments are ways of avoiding our feelings of tension and anxiety – we use them as distractions. But as we become calmer, this is not necessary. Rather than grasping at and holding on to people and situations we simply enjoy them as they are. This does not mean that we become indifferent. In fact, when not driven into situations by anxiety and need we are able to appreciate other people and circumstances for what they are in themselves, rather than as a means of fulfilling our own needs.

Not only does yoga enhance the condition of our nervous system, allowing for improved perception, but as we become calmer our reactions become more measured. As we allow a little spaciousness to develop in our minds we can see more clearly the true nature of people and situations before acting impulsively. This clarity then helps us to discriminate in our daily lives. Our judgement improves. We learn to choose actions, situations, dreams that bring us towards health and happiness. We become conscious of those actions and habits which are self-destructive and unhelpful and, by seeing them for what they are, we let them go.

As we begin to see into the patterns of response with which we meet the world we begin to relax and make friends with ourselves in a very deep way. We accept and acknowledge all aspects of our mind that we have repressed or suppressed. The strength and stability resulting from yoga allow us to integrate what we find without judgement. We no longer have to hide from ourselves and from others. In this acceptance there is a deep sense of peace that is powerful and vibrant, and is expressed in an unshakeable appetite for life. This is true relaxation.

Less and less do we crave for and cling to externals. Instead we find contentment within the circumstances of life as they arise. We do not become complacent or uninterested, but nourish ourselves on the strength we find within. We are no longer troubled by hungers that drive us to the external world for sensory and emotional stimulus. Through enhancing our powers of concentration yoga enhances all of our activities. Often the difference between an activity done well and poorly is simply a matter of whether or not we are paying attention. Consequently all our activities and pursuits improve, bringing a sense of appreciation of our activities and of fulfilment in our lives. Rather then making us disenchanted with the normal round of daily activity, yoga gives us a deeper sense of purpose and fulfilment in our lives as they are.

As this peace and contentment deepen we become happier. Laughter becomes our response to the world, rather than judgement. Contentment leads to calmness; calmness to clarity; clarity to detachment, detachment to contentment. As our awareness deepens inwardly, we discover that the innate oscillation of our nervous system is one of pleasure, of rapture. As our inner awareness strengthens this rapture begins to express itself in our every activity. The joy that we discover through yoga is not dependent on external factors. It is the subtle, inner vibration of our being. It is this that at last begins to satisfy us, providing us with a source of pleasure and joy that can never be taken away. No matter what situation we enter, no matter how ugly or uncomfortable it may appear, with a deep, open quality of awareness we find that it simply acts as a mirror to us. In so doing it reflects back to us the rapturous energy of our inner nervous system. Then the inner and the outer world have become one. We are no longer subject to the tyranny of pain and pleasure, attachment and aversion. We are free to live in the simple ecstasy of being alive.

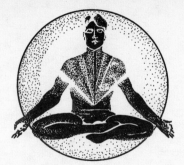

PART 2

THE PRACTICE OF
YOGA SADHANA

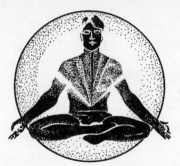

8 · GENERAL GUIDELINES

In Chapter 9 instructions are given for the various yoga postures, breathing exercises and meditation, with suggestions for practice formats at different levels. Read the following guidelines carefully before attempting any of the practices. Although you can use this book to work on your own, it is always beneficial to look for a good yoga instructor to set you on the right path.

There are two kinds of physical discomfort that may be experienced during yoga postures. The first, quite common to begin with or when practising only occasionally, is the natural resistance of under-used muscles to being stretched. This can be felt as an ache or sometimes more powerfully as pain. It is there while stretching, but disappears when you stop. It also comes on gradually, as you extend the muscle, with a consistent smooth quality, increasing or decreasing as you intensify or release the stretch. This discomfort can be worked through with perseverance.

The second kind is the pain of injury. Usually it arises from an old injury being awakened but it can also arise from abusing muscles or joints by over-enthusiastic and insensitive practice. This pain usually arises suddenly and intensely, with a feeling of extreme heat or cold, sharpness or heaviness. It often continues after we release the posture. In order to avoid this, we must always pay close attention to the limits of our muscles and our minds. If we experience pain consistently in a particular posture or group of postures we should seek out an experienced teacher who has a deep and practical understanding of alignment. When the postures are performed without paying attention to alignment the risk of injury is far greater.

If we practise too strenuously or forcefully, we can drain ourselves of energy; conversely, if we practise with attention we generate energy. We must also be wary of laziness in the mind that asks us to stop when there is no need to do so. This occurs not only as a desire to end the practice session early but to release the postures too soon, before the muscles have been fully stretched and held. The best way to time the holding of a posture is by counting breaths. As practice develops we can increase the count for individual postures as we begin to find it easier to hold them.

Progress tends to follow a pattern of plateaux. Initial progress is followed by a period of little improvement, with body and mind adjusting to new possibilities without us noticing. Then all of a sudden this process of assimilation will be complete and we find our capacity for movement has suddenly extended. The cycle then begins again.

Do not judge your progress by your ability to perform and maintain postures; rather, an inner sensitivity to the sensations of freedom and resistance in your body. It is the cultivation of this refined inner sensitivity that bears the richest fruit. To know what we are, to feel what we do, to be in touch with ourselves and the fullness of each moment is both the prize and the process of yoga.

With a regular balanced practice combined with sensible diet (see p. 118–20) your body should establish and maintain its optimum size. This may not dovetail with current cultural assumptions. At the same time that your body is establishing its equilibrium, so also is your mind, and you will come to accept and feel comfortable with your body's particular needs, limitations and possibilities. We are not all genetically primed to be lean, lithe and supple.

If you have any injuries and ailments please consult your doctor before trying any of these postures. People with the following conditions need to take the advice of a trained yoga teacher in order to do yoga postures safely:

Eye and ear problems
M.E.
M.S.
Heart problems
Neck problems
Spinal problems
Recent injuries
Broken or fractured bones
Recent surgery
Pregnancy

PRACTICAL CONSIDERATIONS

Activating the whole body is important in yoga –, how far you move is less important than how you move. Always move with the breath and with awareness of the whole body. To feel and awaken the whole of your body, certain practical principles must be applied.

1. Practise on an empty stomach: three hours after a meal and an hour after a light snack. Wait until the stomach feels empty.
2. Avoid bathing in the half hour before and after practice. Hot and cold showers can oversensitize the muscles and showering immediately after asana can weaken the body by drawing off minerals.
3. When the soles of both feet are on the floor they share the body weight between then – half on one, half on the other. The weight on each foot should be distributed evenly between the heels and the balls of the feet and between the inner and outer edges of the feet. Even placement of the feet is essential to even action of the legs and stable support for the spine.
4. When the legs are straight they should be *straight*, thus allowing the spine to move freely and blood and prana to flow freely in the legs and feet. This is done by pulling up

hard on the kneecaps and then pressing back into the backs of the knees. Pressing back without lifting the kneecaps with the front thigh muscles will only lead to overstretching the backs of the legs.

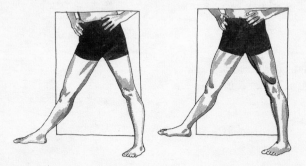

Legs held without quadricep grip   *Quadricep grip*

5. The pelvis should always be level, except when it is deliberately tilted. The sacrum should be kept tucked in and moving up so that the lower back is kept in line without arching. The muscles in the pelvic floor should be contracted and drawn in to protect the lumbar, groin and thigh muscles.

6. The chest should always be kept open by lifting the ribcage up while keeping the shoulders relaxed. At the same time

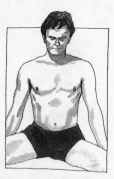
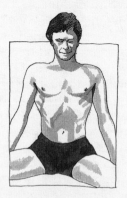

Open chest front: incorrect   *Open chest front: correct*

bring the back ribs, shoulderblades and top spine in towards the front of the body, lifting the side ribs and armpits forward and up.

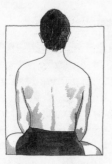

Open chest back: incorrect

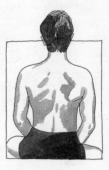

Open chest back: correct

7. The neck should always be a natural extension of the spine, even when turning to the side. Do not allow it to lean in any direction.

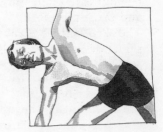

Neck alignment: incorrect

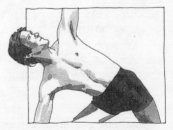

Neck alignment: correct

8. Balance of awareness is needed to maintain balance of action, equalizing the action and the awareness throughout the body. The action in the front of the leg balances the action in the back of the leg. Unbalanced action leads to instability and discomfort. Equally, the action in a posture must be balanced between the top and bottom. So in back bends the action in the spine must be anchored in the action of the legs and the pelvis, and the activity of the spine should be even throughout its entire length.

9. Because the postures are difficult for bodies locked into habitual patterns of imbalance, there is a tendency to strain when in the postures due to too much physical exertion. To avoid this, the postures should be performed with a subtle sensitivity to the responses of each part of the body. The effort is a subtle one of observing and responding throughout the whole body. It is only when the posture becomes effortless that the quality of asana emerges. Then one feels stable, comfortable, light and alive. There should be no tension in the face and throat when in the postures.

10. It is important that yoga is a practice of mind as well as body. Practise with sensitivity and intelligence and be patient and accepting of limitations. The most natural way to progress is to come gently to the existing limit and, quite naturally, that limit – without being forced – extends itself. In this way we gradually and effortlessly become more supple, stronger and more alive.

11. The basic breathing technique described under pranayama should also be practised during asana practice, using the ujaiyi throat action (see p. 107) to slow down and deepen the breath. The breath must not be held when the lungs are full or empty, nor should inhalation or exhalation be broken by pauses. The flow of breath should be smooth and strong, without being harsh or forced.

12. Always use mula bandha (see pp. 54–5) and uddiyana mudra (see p. 57) during asana to protect and stabilize the muscles in the middle of the body. The easiest way to approach this is to use the muscular grips that are needed to simultaneously prevent urination and defecation.

13. In order to gain the maximum benefit from yoga postures, it is advisable to have direct instruction from a teacher trained in the principles of anatomical alignment. Once you have tried the postures in this book and found that you want to develop a regular yoga practice try to find a competent teacher to go to once a week, while maintaining a daily self-practice at home. For further instruction in the proper technique of yoga postures please find your nearest Iyengar Yoga teacher by contacting the Iyengar Yoga Institute.

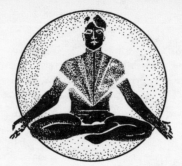

9 · The Postures, Breathing and Meditation

THE STANDING POSTURES

The standing postures are the foundation of safe, effective yoga. They create strength, stability and mobility in the feet, legs, pelvis and spine. Without this the more simple but strenuous backbends, twists and forward bends can overtax the muscles and joints of the body and weaken rather than strengthen them. On a more subtle level the standing postures, due to their complexity, provide the perfect context within which to learn the meditative aspect of asana. In the standing postures the whole body is active, from the feet to the fingers. This activity involves many opposing movements and actions, the establishment and maintenance of which requires a considerable effort of attention. In the simpler, but more strenuous, postures such as backbends it is only too easy to lose complete bodily awareness and become caught in a single part of the body and a peripheral layer of the mind. The standing postures are the indispensable foundation to a well-balanced practice of yoga.

1. RESTING POSE: TADASANA

Stand with feet together. Bear your body weight evenly across the surface of your feet. Keep your legs straight, pull up your kneecaps, stretch your spine up, and open your chest, relaxing your shoulders.

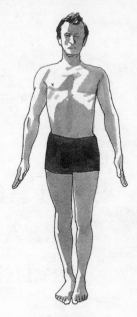

Resting pose

2. MOUNTAIN POSE: URDVAHASTASAN

Stand in resting pose. Stretch your arms up alongside your ears so that your palms face each other and just look up.

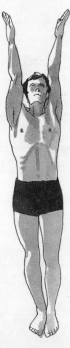

Mountain pose

3. FOLDING POSE: UTTANASAN

Stand in mountain pose. As you exhale bring your arms down in front of you and fold your body in towards your legs, bringing your head in as your lungs empty. Keep legs straight, kneecaps pulled up, weight even on your feet. Relax your neck and shoulders, and take your shoulderblades down your back away from your ears.

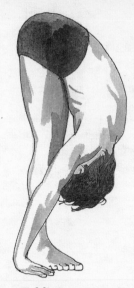

Folding pose

4. RESTING DOG POSE OR DOWNWARD DOG POSE: ADHOMUKHASVANASAN

Lie on the floor, face down, with your hands tucked under your shoulders so you can't see them and your elbows tucked in, keeping your toes tucked under towards the pelvis. As you exhale push back and up on to hands and knees, then stretch and straighten your arms, legs and spine. Pull your kneecaps up, press your legs back, your heels down. Lock your elbows in and roll your shoulders out and up away from your ears. Take your shoulderblades away from your ears and stretch your spine keeping your chest open, lengthening your waist.

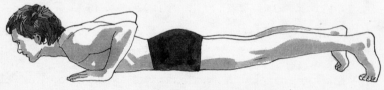

Lying for dog pose

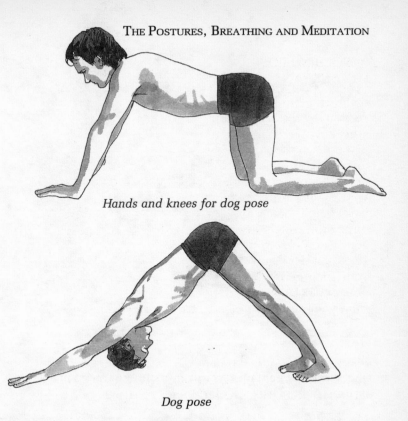

Hands and knees for dog pose

Dog pose

5. TRIANGLE POSE: TRIKONASAN

Stand in resting pose, inhale and extend your arms out from your shoulders parallel to the floor. At the same time jump both feet wide apart so that they come to rest parallel with each other, underneath your wrists. Keep your legs straight and strong, pulling up on the kneecaps. (*See illustration at top of next page*)

6. FOLDED TRIANGLE POSE: PADOTTANASAN

Stand in triangle pose. Exhale and pivot your pelvis forward and down, bringing your fingertips to the floor in line with your shoulders. Bend your arms, lowering your head towards the floor while taking your hands back towards the line of your feet. Press your palms into the floor with your wrists,

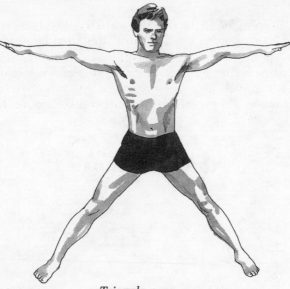

Triangle pose

elbows and shoulders parallel. Make your feet alive and spread your weight on them evenly, pull up on your kneecaps and make your legs straight, long and strong.

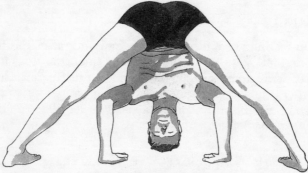

Folded Triangle pose

7. SIDE WARRIOR POSE: PARSVA VIRABADRASAN

Stand in triangle pose, with the feet 4–5 feet apart. Turn the left foot slightly in towards the right and turn the right foot out 90 degrees. Bend the right leg until the thighbone is parallel to the floor, moving the feet until the knee bone is directly above the heelbone, with the buttock bone in line with the knee. Stretch the spine up and open the chest, looking along the right arm as you keep the left leg locked straight and strong while pulling up on the kneecap. Repeat on the other side.

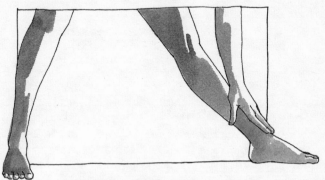

Turning the feet for side warrior pose

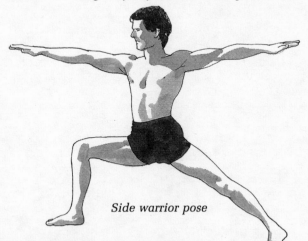

Side warrior pose

8. WARRIOR POSE: VIRABADRASAN

Stand in triangle pose, with the feet 4–5 feet apart. Turn the left foot well in towards the right and turn the right foot out 90 degrees. Turn the pelvis to face directly forwards and

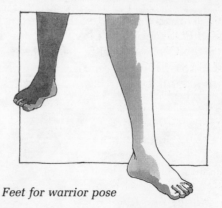

Feet for warrior pose

bend the right leg until the thighbone is parallel to the floor, moving the feet until the knee bone is directly above the heelbone, with the buttock bone in line with the knee. Stretch the spine up and open the chest, looking up along the arms as you keep the left leg locked straight and strong while pulling up on the kneecap. Repeat on the other side.

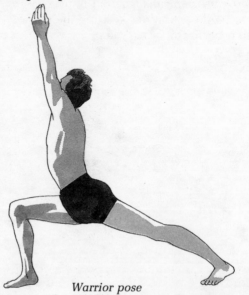

Warrior pose

9. LUNGE AND BOUND LUNGE POSES UTTHITTA PARSVAKONASAN AND PARSVAKONASAN

From triangle pose move into side warrior pose then, stretching forward, bring your ribs along the right thigh, pressing the right hand onto the floor outside the foot, with the arm and leg pressing against each other. Turning the trunk up towards the ceiling look along the left arm towards the hand. Repeat on the other side.

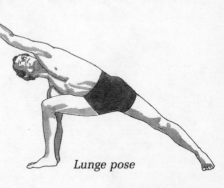

Lunge pose

After holding, change the arms by taking the left arm behind the waist, and feed the right arm through the knee from the front to the back to catch the left hand or wrist. Turn up and look over the left shoulder keeping the spine in line with the thigh. Repeat on the other side.

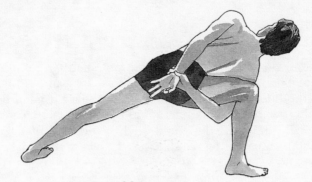

Bound lunge pose

10. SIDE FOLD POSE: PARSVOTTANASAN

From triangle pose with the feet underneath the elbows, turn the left foot well in and the right foot out 90 degrees and turn the pelvis to face straight forwards. With your hands on your hips, stretch the spine up and then pivot the pelvis forward, extending the spine forward and down along the right leg, relaxing the head forward as you come down, hands on either side of the foot. Repeat on the other side.

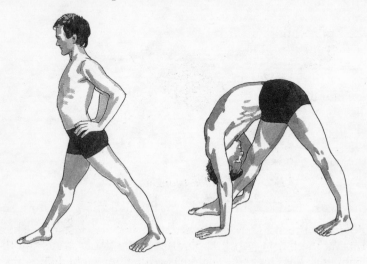

Side fold pose

11. EXTENDED TRIANGLE POSE: UTTHITTA TRIKONASAN

From triangle pose turn the left foot slightly in and the right foot out 90 degrees. Keeping spine long and straight, and without bending at the waist, bring the right hand down the shin towards the ankle by rotating the pelvis like a catherine wheel, and turn the trunk slightly up towards the ceiling looking up at the left hand. Keep the legs both straight, pulling the kneecaps with the front thigh muscles. Repeat on the other side. (*See illustration on top of next page.*)

12. HALF MOON POSE: ARDHACHANDRASAN

Go into the side warrior and then, bringing your weight forwards on to the right foot, stretch your right arm forward and

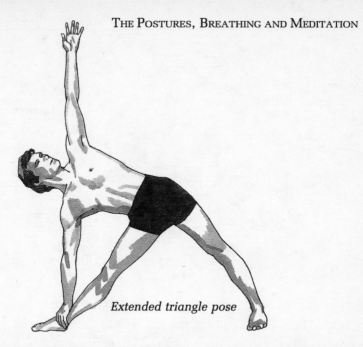

Extended triangle pose

down to the floor as far in front of you as possible. Then, raising the left leg till it is parallel to the floor, straighten the right leg, keeping your balance with your right hand, then turn your trunk up towards the ceiling and look down at the right foot. Keep both legs and the spine straight and long, and roll the left hip and shoulder up as high as you can. Repeat on the other side.

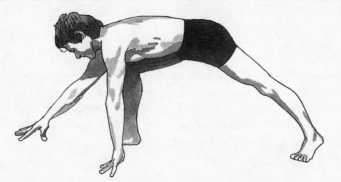

Half moon pose (continued overleaf)

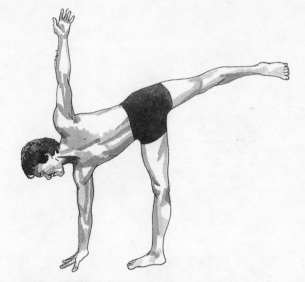

THE FLOOR POSTURES

There are hundreds of floor postures in yoga that, as you progress, work deeper and deeper into every muscle group of the body. The more simple ones are less strenuous than the standing postures and can be used to quiet and cool down body and mind. This can be done after the standing postures, or they can be practised safely on their own to bring about a quietening effect. However, in order to master them safely and effectively, especially the use of the legs, the standing poses must also be practised regularly.

13. STAFF POSE: DANDASAN

Sit on the floor with the legs stretched to the front and pressing together with the inner edges of the feet joined. Press the legs down into the floor and, with the hands cupping the buttocks, fingers pointing to the toes, stretch the spine up, lift the ribcage, open the chest and relax the shoulders looking straight ahead.

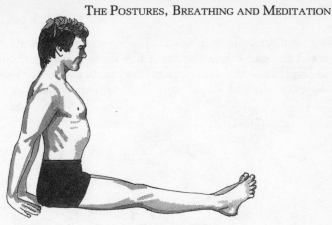

Staff pose

14. HALF LOTUS CYCLE: ARDHAPADMAPASCIMOTTANASAN

Hold each stage of the cycle for from 5–10 breaths.

Stage one. Sit in the staff pose and then place the right foot under the top of the left thigh so the tips of the toes extend beyond the thigh and the heel is in front of the pubic bone. Stretch the spine up, open the chest and then reach forward and catch as far down the left leg as you can while keeping it straight and pressing into the floor with the kneecap pulled up. Catch the foot if you can do so without bending the leg.

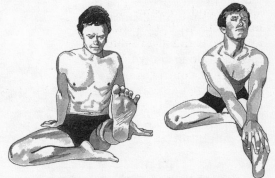

Half lotus cycle: a. Catching the foot   b. Down on leg

Stage two. Keeping hold with the hands, draw the ribcage forwards and lower the chest and head towards or onto your leg, relaxing the neck. Keep the trunk centred, the left leg actively pressing down with the kneecap pulled up.

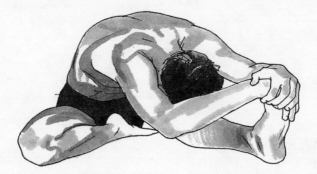

c. Leg on trunk

Stage three. Bring your spine back to a vertical position and hold the right foot or leg in front of you so that the leg is straight. Stretch the spine up, lift the ribcage and open the chest, keeping the right leg relaxed, the left leg straight. Look up.

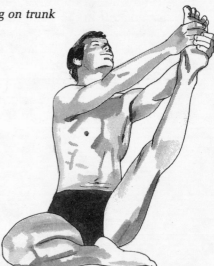

d. Leg up in air, active

Stage four. Holding your left heel or leg in your left hand take it to the left, while turning your head to the right. Stretch the spine up, lift the ribcage and open the chest, with your right hand on your right hip.

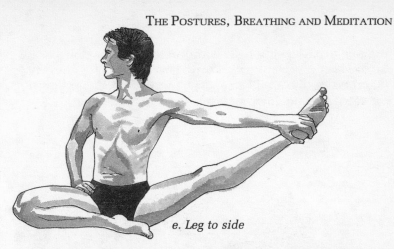

e. Leg to side

Stage five. Bring your left leg back to the centre and hold the foot in your right hand, putting the left hand on the left hip. Straighten the leg and take it across your body to the right while turning your trunk away to the left. Stretch the spine up, lift the ribcage and open the chest.

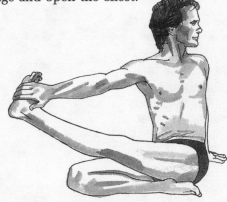

f. Twisting

Stage six. Repeat on the other side.

15. FULL FORWARD BEND: PASCIMOTTANASAN

Sit in the staff pose. Stretch your spine up and reach forward to catch as far down your legs as you can, holding your feet if possible; keep your legs straight. Lift the spine and ribs up, pressing your legs down. Then, keeping the length in your waist, extend forwards and down towards or onto your legs. Relax your neck, shoulders and spine, but keep the legs pressing down into the floor with the kneecaps pulled up.

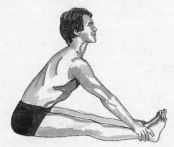

Full forward bend

16. BOAT POSE: NAVASAN

Sit in the staff pose. Place your hands near your knees, pressing your fingertips into the floor and then, leaning back slightly, raise both legs off the floor keeping them straight and pressing the feet together. If you can, raise your arms parallel to the floor alongside your knees. Lift your legs and spine as high as you can, raising the ribcage and opening the chest. Look straight ahead.

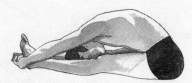

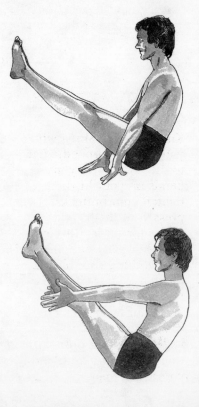

Boat pose

17. RAMP POSE: PURVOTTANASAN

Sit in the staff pose and place your hands 8–12 inches behind you with your fingers pointing forwards. Pressing your hands down, straighten your arms, and with your legs strong and feet pressing together, lift your pelvis as high as you can. Lifting your ribcage up and opening your chest, slowly lengthen your neck and take your head back and down towards your shoulders.

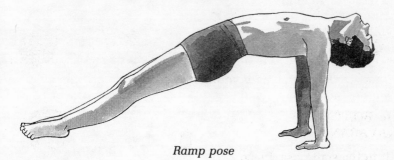

Ramp pose

18. HALF CAMEL POSE: ARDHUSTRASAN

Kneel on your shins with your thighs perpendicular to the floor. With your hands on your hips, tighten your buttocks, press your thighs and pelvis forwards, lift your ribcage, open your chest and, arching your back as much as you can, slowly lengthen your neck and take your head back and down towards your shoulders Keep your thighs perpendicular and your chest open.

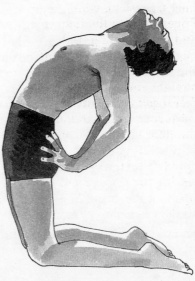

Half camel pose

93

19. TWISTING POSE: PARVRITASAN

Sit in the staff pose. Draw the knees up and your feet halfway in towards you and wrap your arms around your knees, pressing them together. Take your right arm around behind you in line with your left buttock, and bring your

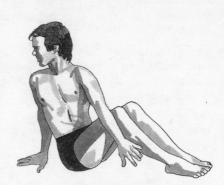

Twisting pose

left arm across your body and press it back against your right knee, pushing back with your knees so they do not move. Lift your spine and chest and turn to your right, looking over your right shoulder. Repeat on the other side.

20. SUPINE TWIST: SUPTAIKAPADAPARVRITASAN

Lie on your back with your arms outstretched and raise the left knee up, placing your left foot on the floor against the inner right knee. Keeping the left foot hooked behind the right knee, roll over on to your right hip and ribs as far as you can and turn your head to look at your left hand. Keep both shoulders close to the floor, legs and spine relaxed. Open your chest and stretch your hands away from each other pressing them and your shoulders into the floor. Repeat on the other side.

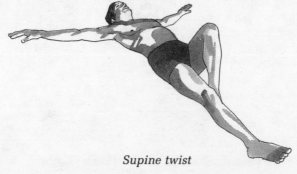

Supine twist

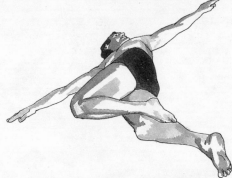

THE FINISHING SEQUENCE

To slowly quieten the mind and body and prepare for relaxation, always finish your practice with the following sequence of postures. Although the whole sequence can be done on its own, do not do any of the postures on their own, with the exception of the half shoulderstand or the half fish.

21. HALF SHOULDERSTAND: ARDHASARVANGASAN

Lie on your back with arms, legs and spine long, chest open. Raise your legs, then lift your pelvis a little off the floor and place your palms under your buttocks, not your back. Take the weight of your legs on your palms so they are at a 90 degree angle from your body and press your shoulders and elbows into the floor, opening your chest by lifting the upper spine up into the chest. **Caution: This pose should be avoided during menstruation**.

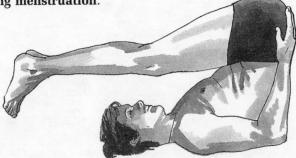

Half shoulderstand (Continued overleaf)

95

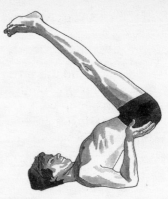

22. PLOUGH POSE: HALASAN

From the half shoulderstand roll up and over on to the tops of your shoulders, taking the tips of the toes to the floor behind your head while keeping your legs straight. Keep the waist and spine long, lifting the pelvis away from the face. For those who cannot reach the floor in the plough, place a stool, box, or some other firm support behind your head when you lie down for half shoulderstand so you can rest your toes on it rather than trying to bring them to the floor. **Caution: this pose should be avoided during menstruation**.

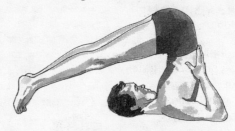

Plough pose

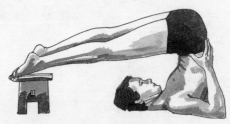

Plough on box

23. EMBRYO POSE: KARNAPIDASAN

From the plough pose, bend your legs bringing your knees towards the floor beside your ears. Relax your feet, legs, hips and spine. If you cannot bring your knees down to the floor, then place them either on your arms or your forehead.

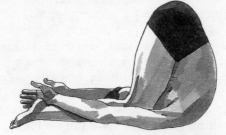

Embryo pose   a. Knees down

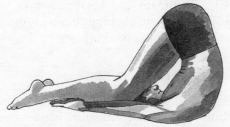

b. Knees on arms

24. SHOULDERSTAND: SARVANGASAN

From the embryo pose, straighten your legs, support your back and walk your feet as close to your face as you can, then lift your legs up in the air keeping them straight. Stretch up from your shoulders into your legs in as straight a line as possible, lifting the spine

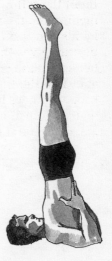

Shoulderstand

and ribcage up away from the floor, with your legs straight and lifting themselves upwards. Use your hands to support and lift your back as close to your shoulderblades as possible. To finish roll down to the floor slowly and gently. **Caution: This pose should be avoided during menstruation**.

25. HALF FISH POSE: ARDHAMATSYASAN

From the staff pose lean back onto your elbows. Press your legs together and into the floor and, arching your back, lift your chest as high as you can. Opening your chest as much as possible, slowly lengthen your neck and take your head back and down towards your shoulders. Keep lifting your chest to take the weight of your head away from the neck and onto the spine and chest.

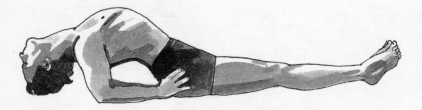

Half fish pose

26. RELAXATION POSE: SAVASANA OR 'CORPSE'

To finalize your practice and harmonize body and mind before pranayama and meditation, finish by doing the relaxation

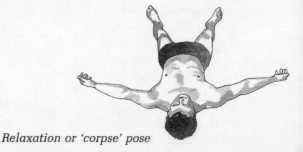

Relaxation or 'corpse' pose

pose. Whenever you do asana or pranayama do relaxation pose for from five to fifteen minutes. It can also be done on its own as an effective form of stress management and relaxation.

To create deep relaxation in the muscles each muscle group in the body has to be systematically released. This is done in two ways: either by going through the body and tensing each muscle group and then releasing in turn, or simply by taking your attention systematically through every part of your body and allowing it to soften. Rather than tensing the muscles, you just allow yourself to feel each part of the body softening, opening and releasing. In both cases, you feel the muscles release the muscular tissues will lengthen and open. This can be felt in a gentle sinking of the bones downwards towards the floor. This is because gravity is no longer resisted by muscular tension and the bones are now more prone to its pull. After a while the general feeling throughout the whole body is one of lightness and openness.

You may find that some areas resist you. Perhaps the tension will not release; perhaps you find that you cannot make clear contact with the muscles in that part. First release all the surrounding muscle groups that you can. Then, gradually and patiently with no hurry or strain, allow the surrounding softness and lightness to spread into the tense or dull area. The throat and face muscles in particular – of which there are over one hundred – can resist, so spend plenty of time allowing them to do so. You are trying to relax and this will only happen if you are patient and sensitive. If you try to force it, or become anxious, you will only become more tense.

When you have released the whole body, keep your attention focused on the sensations in your body openly, without evaluation. You may notice the beating of your heart and then the rise and fall of your chest or abdomen as you breathe. You may feel tingling sensations in your limbs or rumblings in your belly. Become acquainted with the activities inside your body as you relax. By paying close, but relaxed, attention to the activity of the body the mind is no longer able to cling to its patterns of anxiety and worry; it too begins to relax. This is a vital part of the process and is lost if we simply indulge in daydreaming, or thinking, once we have released all physical tension.

The sequence is to soften the face and brain and then take the softness through the whole of your body to the tips of the fingers and the tips of the toes. Go slowly and methodically, trying to feel each muscle group releasing, and even every individual muscle. Repeat the sequence a number of times to make sure that each part of your body has released fully. Each time you do you will feel more relaxed, more open.

When you release the face and head, feel your senses turning inwards. Allow your eyes and ears to melt down into your brain. Feel your nose and throat, your tongue and palate softening and melting. When the senses are no longer turned outwards it is much easier for the brain and the mind to relax. Do not get up until your breath and heartbeat have become soft and smooth. Get up slowly, awakening your body gradually, and roll on to your right side to come up.

SITTING POSTURES

In all the following sitting postures, used for pranayama and meditation, the action in the trunk and spine is the same. The hands can rest on the knees, thighs or lap. Because the lotus posture gives the greatest stability it is the favoured posture, but any of the others will do until the lotus becomes comfortable. In order to achieve the greatest stability it is important to keep the knees below the hips. For some this will mean using blankets, cushions or blocks under the buttocks so the knees rest easily on the floor. In this case sit with the buttock bones to the front edge of the support so that the top of the pelvis is very slightly tilted forwards.

STRETCHING THE SPINE IN SITTING POSTURES

Sucking the perineum into the pelvis, press the sacrum in, tilting the hipbones slightly forwards. Stretch the whole spine up and extend the waist evenly on both sides, lifting the ribcage and the armpits forward and up. Soften the diaphragm and open the floating ribs. Draw the back ribs in and lift the breastbone. Allow the

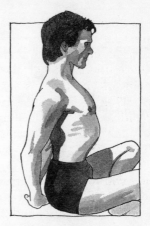

Stretching the spine in sitting postures

shoulders to move back as the chest opens. Allow the shoulder-blades to move down towards the waist.

HERO POSE: VIRASAN

Sit down with the knees bent back so the buttocks rest on the floor in between the heels. If the buttocks do not reach the floor, place a small cushion under them so as to prevent strain at the knee and ankle. Stretch through the ankles so that the line of the foot is an extension of the shin. Place the heels of the hands on the outer

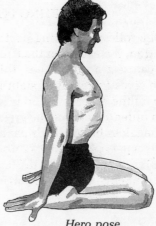

Hero pose

edges of the feet and press them down. At the same time press the outer ankles inwards. Both of these actions should help the inner thighs to lift and bring the tops of the knees parallel to the floor. Keep the knees down and together.

EASY POSE: SUKASAN

Sit on the floor with the legs in front. Draw the left leg in under the right thigh. Cross the right shin under the left. Draw the right foot under the left thigh. This is the most simple cross legged position and can be done on both sides.

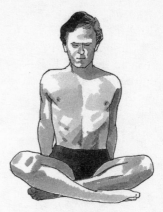

Easy pose

ACCOMPLISHED POSE: SIDASAN

Sit with the legs in front. Bend the left leg and place the heel near the perineum so the sole of the foot rests against the right thigh. Bend the right leg and place the right ankle over the left ankle so the right heel rests against the pubis. Do not sit on the heels. An easy variation is to place

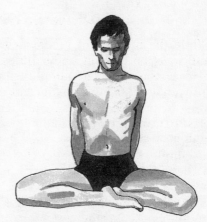

Accomplished pose

the right foot in front of the left so that the heel rests just above the ankle. This is known as the Burmese pose.

LOTUS POSTURE: PADMASAN

Sit in the staff pose. Carefully lift the right foot and, releasing the flesh of the calf, pull the heel into its own groin so that the calf and thigh are tight together. Draw the right thigh towards the left, gently lifting the right foot on to the left thigh as high as it will go. The sole of the foot should face the ceiling. Do

not pull on the knee.
Carefully lift the left foot
and pull the heel into its
own groin so that the calf
and thigh are tight
together. Gently lift and
place the left foot at the
root of the right thigh, the
foot facing up. Carefully
draw the inner thighs
towards each other.

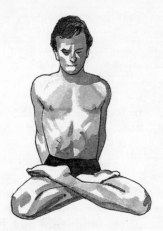

Full lotus

PRANAYAMA

While the practice of pranayama is profound and complex
and must be learned under the guidance of an experienced
teacher, the basics are simply learning how to use the lungs
fully. In order to enhance the capacity of the lungs pranayama
must be prepared for by asana, which not only develops the
elasticity and resilience of the lung tissue but also strengthens
and purifies the nervous system. It takes considerable practice
of simple inhalation and exhalation to prepare lungs and
nerves for the alternate nostril and retention techniques of
pranayama. So, to be safe, we proceed very slowly and cau-
tiously, learning first the mechanical techniques for developing the lungs and the correct actions of inhalation and exhalation.

The breath can be divided into three separate phases:
diaphragmatic, thoracic and clavicular. Many people only use
either the diaphragmatic/abdominal phase or the thoracic
phase. Very few use both of them. Fewer still ever use the
clavicular phase. This is not only because our sedentary life-
styles do not require vast amounts of oxygen but also because
of emotional tension.

Because of this, learning to activate the lungs fully in all
three phases can initially be difficult. The brain may be confused by the activation of dormant lung tissue. Releasing of

emotional tension that was locked into frozen lung tissue may create resistance. If either breathlessness or feelings of panic occur, pause and allow your breath to return to normal before continuing. If it persists, then postpone your practice till a later date, perhaps after having worked more deeply with your practice of asana – savasana in particular.

In the complete breath, fill and empty the lungs as we would any vessel, such as a jar. Fill from the bottom to the top, and empty from the top to the bottom. Because the breath and our emotional state are connected, make the breath as soft and smooth as possible as this quietens the mind. Breathe slowly and with care so that the sound of the breath remains soft and fluid, keeping a constant consistency and flowing evenly from outbreath to inbreath. When learning the full activation of the complete breath do not count the length of inhalation and exhalation. This can be done after we have mastered the mechanical technique. To have mastered the breath means that we can, repeatedly and at will, breathe fully and deeply in and out of our lungs with a soft, smooth, consistent rhythm, activating the lungs consciously in the desired sequence. This technique alone can take many years of daily practice to master.

By learning the complete breath – activating the diaphragm, the thoracic lung and the clavicular lung – we not only absorb more oxygen and expel more carbon dioxide but we also absorb more prana, developing reserves of energy which can enhance the physical, emotional and mental creativity of our lives. We can only absorb as much prana as our lungs can expand to take in. As our lungs gain in elasticity and strength, they open more and allow in more prana.

Breath retention, however, does not have this built-in balancing mechanism. By holding the breath in our lungs for an extended period, the blood not only absorbs more oxygen through the alveoli, it also absorbs more prana, regardless of how well the lungs have been activated. By holding the breath we can absorb more prana into our system than the system is ready for. This should be avoided. However, if we proceed gradually, mastering inhalation and exhalation, by the time we get to retention our lungs and nerves will be well prepared.

Pranayama should be practised in a sitting posture at least once a day for ten minutes or more. Ideally it should be practised on its own, or after asana practice. If practising after asanas, be sure to rest first in savasana until the heart and respiration become tranquil and the nerves quiet.

Also, be careful to respect the capacity of your lungs and nerves on a daily basis. Any strain in the lungs or pressure in the head, eyes or ears indicates that the lungs or brain are being over-taxed. If this arises, cease practice for the day and rest in savasana.

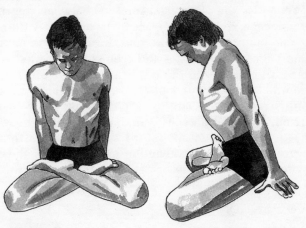

Deep inhalation, seen from front (a) and side (b)

INHALATION OR PURAKA

Take up one of the sitting positions outlined above. Exhale deeply, expelling the air from the bottom of the lungs by drawing in the abdominal muscles. Maintaining a gentle grip on the abdominal muscles begin to inhale slowly and smoothly through the nostrils. Allow air to enter the bottom of the lungs so that the diaphragm begins to move down towards the navel. As the diaphragm lowers, pressure will begin between the force of this action and that of the grip you have on your abdominal muscles. Maintain your grip so this gentle pressure remains throughout inhalation. It should not create strain. This grip not only prevents the abdomen from distending, it also helps to anchor the lungs so that they do not rise as you try to fill the top lung, thereby reducing the capacity of your inhalation. As the lower lung fills allow the breath to rise evenly into the thoracic lungs so that the floating ribs begin to open and lift. You do not have to do this deliberately; as your lungs fill it will happen automatically. When the floating ribs have lifted and opened allow the air to fill the upper lung evenly on the left and right and front and back. The upper chest and breast bone should rise gradually until the collar bones lift up and it feels as if the air is coming into your throat. Use the intercostal muscles between the ribs to raise the ribcage, giving more space to the opening of the upper lung.

For many people conscious inhalation is extremely difficult. It can take months and even years to perfect – especially breathing fully into the upper lung and maintaining the abdominal grip throughout. However, patient practice is the only way to success for forcing the lungs can be dangerous. If dizziness, breathlessness, anxiety, pressure in eyes, ears or head are experienced, return to normal breathing and try again. If they persist, abandon pranayama for the day. These symptoms will not necessarily occur the next time.

EXHALATION OR RECHAKA

As the lungs fill to capacity on complete inhalation, take a gentle grip on your chest muscles. This will help to keep the act of exhalation smooth and consistent. Allow the upper lung to empty by letting go of the upper intercostal muscles one by one, from the collar bones downwards. In the beginning this is almost impossible and

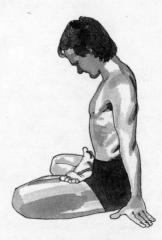

Full exhalation

you will find that the whole of the upper chest releases as one. With time and practice you will be able to isolate the different bands of intercostal muscles more easily and the action will become more gradual and more smooth. Then allow the floating ribs to move downwards and towards each other as the air leaves the middle lung. When the floating ribs can move no lower, allow the air to be pushed out of the lower lung by the diaphragm rising. To complete this action draw the abdominal muscles in tightly so that the viscera force the diaphragm upwards.

Full exhalation, like full inhalation, is very difficult. The aim is to learn to release the intercostal muscles one by one consciously so that exhalation is gradual and smooth. At first this will be impossible and the whole chest will release at once. To release one must develop conscious control of muscles that are habitually unconscious. Patience and sensitivity are vital. If a feeling of breathlessness arises before exhalation is complete do not fight it. Let go of the action you are working on and allow a few normal breaths; then, following a deep exhalation, return to your practice on an inhalation. Do not attempt to hurry to your deepest breath. Allow the transition from normal breathing to full breathing to be very gradual so as to avoid straining the lungs.

ADVANCED VARIATIONS

The following techniques allow for a more complete inhalation and exhalation.

Ujaiyi

This is done by very gently contracting the inner lower muscles of the throat so that it narrows. The action is rather like the beginning of swallowing when you can feel the front of the throat moving towards the back. This narrowing of the throat naturally slows down the passage of air in and out of the lungs, allowing more control to be exerted which will maintain smoothness and ensure a complete inhalation and exhalation.

Mula bandha

During inhalation and exhalation activate mula bandha. This is done by contracting the anal and urogenital muscles. When the anal muscles are contracted it feels as if you are trying to prevent elimination from the bowel; when the urogenital muscles are contracted it feels as though you are trying to prevent elimination from the bladder.

Quietness

The effort to keep the breath quiet requires subtle control of the muscular action of inhalation and exhalation. This control helps to maintain smoothness and consistency.

Length

The length of breath refers to the force rather than duration of the breath. In exhalation this is measured by the distance away from the nostrils at which the breath can still be felt. By shortening the length of breath until it cannot even be felt leaving the nose, again one must take complete control of the muscular actions which create the slow, soft, smooth and consistent breath. Traditionally one exhales so as not to disturb a feather placed under the nostrils.

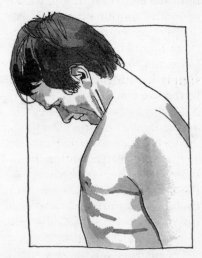

Jalandhara bandha

This is done by pressing the chin onto the breastbone. It is learned through practice of the shoulders and and should not be forced. The throat must be kept passive, and attention must be paid to

Jalandhara bandha

the neck muscles to ensure they are not straining. Jalandhara bandha relaxes the upper lung tissue and therefore lessens resistance to the final phase of the complete breath. These methods all help to bring the ind more directly into contact with the breath. By uniting our awareness with the action of our breath, which is smooth and calm, our mind also becomes tranquil and peaceful. A mind without tension and anxiety has energy available for clear perception and lucid thought. This is a necessary precursor to the subtle awareness of mental processes awakened in meditation.

MEDITATION

The basic purpose of meditation is to develop the tone and capacity of our mind. Memory, analysis, perception, inference, concentration, recognition, recall are all like muscles which we need to keep in trim if they are to serve us well. As our minds are our most valuable asset, which we use constantly to guide and direct our lives, the importance of meditation as a means to improving the quality of our lives cannot be over-emphasized.

By concentrating on a seed that has little interest for our minds we develop the capacity to remain more deeply concentrated on our normal daily activities. By becoming more deeply concentrated when going about our daily tasks we do them more effectively. This concentration – that we practise in meditation and that carries over into our daily life – is quite simply learning to keep both mind and body focused together in the same activity. When they are not in conflict with each other their co-operation leads to a more efficient use of energy and more skilful and effective action.

Most of the so-called meditation techniques taught today are in fact concentration techniques. Concentration can be practised, whereas meditation is a spontaneous process. As the mind becomes more and more focused and unified through concentration, the usual disturbances that assault the mind drop away: when the mind becomes quiet, then a state of meditation emerges.

For many people sitting meditation is too difficult and it is easier to experience meditation or absorption in asana. The inner awareness of alignment and freedom within an asana becomes the seed which absorbs the mind, quietening it, and allowing a sense of peace and vitality to emerge spontaneously. Sitting meditation then becomes an extension of asana practice, in which the line and stability of the posture are vital to the process of quietening the mind. The stronger and more stable our sitting posture, the deeper will be our concentration. In this way asana is a preparation for meditation. Similarly, the concentration required to master the mechanical techniques of pranayama prepare the mind for the deeper, more abstract concentration of meditation.

Even those with weak or stiff spines can practise meditation using a bench or a chair. Meditation has many benefits which can be reaped long before deep one-pointedness occurs. These

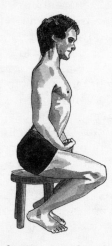

Meditating on a bench

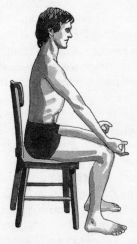

Meditating on a chair

benefits result from the close and uncensored observation of our mental and emotional processes which occurs when we spend time watching our mind trying to become focused on a seed. They include improved concentration, enhanced recall, increased clarity of perception, emotional stability, improved judgement, perseverance and determination, improved self-knowledge, enhanced self-esteem.

While there are many techniques for the practice of meditation, they all embody one guiding principle. This is the use of a seed to narrow the activity of the mind to a single point. Outlined below are the four basic seeds used in many schools of meditation. They are given in order of progressive difficulty.

The breath should not be manipulated, but there should be a light downward grip on the abdominal muscles so as to focus physical and psychic energy in the lower abdomen. Before starting, decide how long you will sit and do not stop until that time has passed. In the beginning it is better to choose a shorter time. Then, as practice deepens, it can be extended. Remember not to move unless absolutely necessary – moving the feet, itching, or twitching the nose will all dissipate the energy of concentration that you have accumulated. It is the energy that you accumulate through concentration that allows your awareness to cut deeper into the patterns of your mind.

Each of the following methods should be practised in a strong, stable sitting posture with spine straight and chest open. The hands can rest on the thighs, knees or lap, or they may be held in one of the mudras.

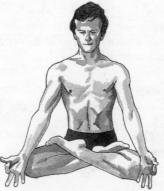

Meditating with a mudra

Counting inhalation and exhalation

Beginning on an exhalation count one. On the inhalation count two. On the exhalation count three. Continue up to ten. If you reach ten return to one again, or if you lose count or your mind wanders, also return to one.

Counting exhalations

Practise as with the previous exercise but counting only the outbreath. This is harder because to go from one count to the next takes longer.

Counting inhalations

Practise as with the previous exercise but counting only the inbreath. This is harder still because the outbreath is the phase of relaxation and, on the inbreath the mind tends to wander more easily.

Following the breath

Simply follow the breath without counting. Feel the breath moving in and out of the lower abdomen, uniting with your mental concentration and the concentration of your physical energy. Observe, without interference, the natural flow of breath in and out, and the physical and energetic quality of your posture.

It is sometimes helpful to spend a short while at the beginning of a meditation period simply observing the body and the mind. This should be done with no attempt at control, interference or judgement. Begin by openly observing the sensations of your body, without reacting or analysing. Feel the quality of contact between your legs and the floor; the sensation of your spine; the feel of your shoulders. Likewise allow the mind to go where it will and observe this movement without prejudice or judgement. Then as the mind naturally begins to settle begin to practise whichever concentration technique you are working with. Too much force is counter-productive. The mind is rather like a wild stallion: if you tie it to a post it will rebel and break free and escape beyond your control; if, however, you give it a meadow to roam in, it will settle down and become peaceful. It is important to be patient and gradual in your practice of meditation.

SELF-PRACTICE: YOGA SADHANA

The techniques of asana, pranayama and samyama should be learned gradually and gently. It is better to do a short practice regularly than a longer one occasionally. Postures can be repeated a number of times while they are being learned and not held for long. Initially, if you find the postures unfamiliar, confusing or uncomfortable hold them only for one or two breaths and then repeat them two or three times. Once they have become comfortable you can hold them longer. Even a very short daily practice will bring benefits. This alone will bring improvement in respiration, muscle tone, flexibility and stamina. After a while you will find that you want to increase the amount of time you give to your yoga practice. Then you can begin to work through the following practice formats:

1. BEGINNER'S PRACTICE LEVEL

Resting Pose	79
Mountain Pose	79
Folding Pose	80
Dog Pose	81
Staff Pose	89
Half Lotus Cycle	89
Twisting Pose	94
Finishing Sequence	95–98
Relaxation Pose	98
Pranayama	103–105

2. INTERMEDIATE PRACTICE LEVEL

Resting Pose	79
Mountain Pose	79
Folding Pose	80
Dog Pose	81
Triangle Pose	82
Folding Pose	80
Side Warrior	83
Warrior	84

Floor Postures
(in the order given in the text)   88–94
Finishing Sequence   95–98
Relaxation Pose   98
Pranayama   103–105

3. ADVANCED PRACTICE LEVEL

All Standing Postures
(in the order given in the text)   78–87
Floor Postures
(in the order given in the text)   88–94
Finishing Postures   95–98
Relaxation Pose   98
Pranayama   103–105
Meditation   109–112

4. SPECIAL PRACTICE FOR EVENINGS WHEN TIRED

Floor Postures   88–94
Finishing Postures   95–98
Relaxation Pose   98
Pranayama   103–105

5. SPECIAL PRACTICE FOR QUIETENING AND CALMING

Finishing Sequence   95–98
Relaxation Pose   98
Pranayama   103–105
Meditation   109–112

6. SPECIAL SHORT PRACTICE FOR QUIETENING AND CALMING

Relaxation Pose   98
Pranayama   103–105
Meditation   109–112

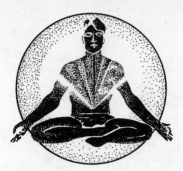

PART 3

YOGA AS A WAY OF LIFE

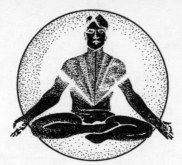

10 · YOGA AND DAILY LIFE

Yoga has not survived five thousand years without good reason. While many people imagine that it has always been an esoteric, marginal activity confined to a small minority this is not the case. Yoga, in one form or another, has permeated the cultures of the Far East for millennia. Not only in India, but also in Burma, Thailand and South-East Asia, Tibet, Nepal, China and Japan, yoga has been a vital part of the fabric of daily life. Yoga probably still has a greater effect on these countries than Christianity has in the modern West.

Yoga is available in many forms, which include teaching for all the different paths. However, the great and increasing popularity of yoga rests upon its universal and perennial adaptability. The modern world is witnessing a new, secular development in yoga. Many modern yogis have adapted their tradition to make yoga – especially asana, pranayama and meditation – more accessible to industrial society. The techniques are being taught piecemeal without their traditional philosophical framework. Yoga is – even in such a fragmentary, secular package – a system of physical, mental and spiritual wellbeing that has no equal in any culture. It offers fitness, health, confidence, concentration, clarity, calmness, generosity, openness and many more benefits that can enrich the lives of each and every one of us. Once it has been experienced the power of yoga is something that soon becomes the foundation of a challenging, creative and satisfying life.

YOGA AND FAMILY

The most influential of modern yogis is undoubtedly the late Krishnamacharya of Mysore. Not only was he a family man with children but so also are all three of his most influential students: B. K. S. Iyengar of Pune, K. Pattabhi Jois of Mysore and T. S. Desikachar of Madras. Being celibate and without a family has never been necessary for yoga. Fitting yoga into family life is simply a matter of priorities. It soon becomes obvious that time given to yoga is not lost to other family members or obligations because of its beneficial effects. One simple result of yoga practice is to induce better sleep, which often means that the time taken to do yoga can be taken from time spent in bed. By rising half an hour early and doing yoga instead of sleeping, and even retiring half an hour later and doing half an hour in the evening, the end result will be more not less energy. In addition, the effect of yoga on the nervous system and the mind tends to make us more efficient in our everyday activities which often means that we spend less time doing the daily chores than we did previously because our minds are focused and we pay better attention to what we are doing. Along with increased energy yoga creates a state of relaxation, openness and adaptability that can only enhance family life.

YOGA AND FOOD

Yoga has always placed great emphasis on the food that is conducive to progress. Yogis recognized that the quality of our consciousness is to a great extent determined by what we eat, since this determines the quality of our blood, which determines the quality of every cell in our body including our central nervous system. This in turn affects the quality of our perceptions and therefore our mood.

Consequently, yoga texts categorize foods into those we should and should not eat to enhance our yoga practice. This categorization is based on the concept of the three gunas, which are the basic energies or qualities that underlie all existence. *Sattva* promotes clarity and luminosity; *rajas* creates energy and strength; *tamas* creates inertia or heaviness. Some yoga texts stress more sattvic foods, while others prefer more rajasic foods.

The purpose of food is nourishment, however. Rather than choosing food from habit or on the basis of taste, we should choose foods that will develop strength, vitality and sensitivity. This means eating natural, seasonal, organic, locally grown foods whenever possible. They should be whole and un-adulterated, mainly composed of whole grains, a wide range of vegetables and fruits, nuts, seeds, and occasional dairy products. Avoid bitter, acid, salty, pungent, spicy, stale, highly processed and reheated foods.

When using traditional yogic guidelines it is important to recognize that individual foods should be appropriate to the climate in which you live. Many of the foods associated with yoga are native to India, which has a very specific climate. To eat a diet suited to India would not work as well in colder, wetter, temperate climates which have four or five seasons rather than three. Another consideration is that the effect of individual foods is changed by combining them with other foods.

The best way to adapt your diet to help your yoga practice is to listen to your body. As your practice develops so will your sensitivity to foods. Those foods that make you dull and heavy (tamasic) or tense and overexcitable (rajasic) will begin to lose their appeal, while those that make you calm and clear (sattvic) will attract you. Imposing strict rules of diet never works. Allow your own practice and your own body to guide you gently towards a nourishing diet. In general, animal foods create tension and insensitivity, while dairy products create dullness and softness. Dairy products are therefore sometimes useful as a buffer against intense, impetuous practice, especially of pranayama, which can lead to hypersensitivity of the nervous system. Grains create strength and stamina, but in excess create heaviness and inertia. Vegetables provide lightness and mobility, but in excess create weakness. Fruits create softness and flexibility but in excess create unsteadiness. Salt in moderation creates clarity, strength and flexibility; in excess it creates hardness and stagnation. Sugar creates confusion, excitement and hypersensitivity leading to insensitivity, but in tiny amounts can create relaxation. One essential guiding principle of diet is that quantity changes quality.

YOGA AND SEX

Yoga and sex are inextricable. The practice of yoga reveals the single continuum of human nature. It is not possible to separate sexual energy from anatomical, physiological, emotional, mental or spiritual energy. Yoga can be understood as a process of transforming sexual energy into spiritual energy, but this transformation does not involve the denial of sexual energy. To progress in yoga we have to establish a new, unconditioned, creative expressiveness of our sexuality. The further we advance along the spiritual path of yoga the less this creative expression resembles the compulsive, habitual patterns of sexual behaviour to which we have been conditioned.

The sex drive is a powerful, natural and necessary appetite. It cannot be healthily denied, but must be released and channelled consciously. On each of the different paths of yoga the means to do this vary, but in those yogas that are inherently tantric – that honour and utilize the body – the methods are similar. They start by awakening and strengthening the body, which inevitably awakens our sexual energy as a result of regeneration of the sexual organs and an increase in general vitality. Long before the kundalini itself awakens, the energy of muladhara chakra begins to leak into the system if aswini mudra and mula bandha (see pp. 54–5) have not been perfected. This leakage, if it is not recognized, can lead to difficulties and confusion that can hinder and even arrest further progress: these can include excessive sexual desire, extreme sexual potency and unconscious sexual manipulation. It is therefore important to practice mula bandha, aswini mudra and vajroli mudra (see p. 57) from the outset. As they are difficult to master, do not rush into more advanced practice of asana and pranayama until you feel confident that you are adequately prepared.

The tantric yogas – Hatha Yoga and Kundalini Yoga in particular – are designed to approach this problem head on. In Hatha Yoga texts the sex act is openly referred to and techniques are given to use it creatively. In Tantra Yoga itself the emphasis is on conscious sexual activity that awakens the physical and subtle body, generating and focusing energy that can then be used spiritually for illumination and liberation. One of the requirements is the guidance of a guru to ensure that we do not become caught in destructive sexuality. The main safeguards are the perfection of mula bandha, pranayama, and meditation. Mula bandha helps to keep the energies of mula dhara focused and contained and eventually, with the help of uddiyana bandha (see p. 55), directed upwards. Pranayama provides the tranquillity to remain unperturbed by strong sexual feelings. The depth and clarity of meditation afford the opportunity to recognize the source and consequences of these feelings and to see through the ways we distort them destructively. Through these special techniques sexual energy is brought under conscious control and is then directed towards spiritual awakening.

For most yoga students the effect of their practice on their sexuality is positive and wholesome. As they become healthier, more alive and more self-confident, this spills over into every aspect of their lives, including sexuality. An increase in sexual appetite, sensitivity and stamina is a happy outcome of yoga practice rather than a hindrance. But even in these instances sexual activity is not necessarily a hindrance. It is the underlying motivation and intention that matters.

CONCLUSION

In its effect yoga is a systematic, gradual process of relaxation. First, through the postures, we relax physical tension. This physical release brings about at the same time a release of emotional trauma, because emotions that we do not allow ourselves to feel fully as they arise tend to become repressed and are stored in the tissues of muscles and organs as physical hardness. By doing the yoga asana we release this hardness, in both muscles and organs, and with that the emotional tension held there is also released.

In order to master the art of smooth, deep inhalation and exhalation complete control must be established over all the muscles of the throat and chest – they must become completely free from tension so they will move freely and fully. This is begun in the asana, especially in backward movements of the spine, and refined in pranayama. As these muscles become free from hardness they release their associated emotional stagnation. This is usually related to feelings of love and trust and their communication. As the muscles of the chest begin to release, so our emotional centre – the heart – begins to open. We let go of our fears of intimacy and self-expression. This makes us not only more open and able to love and trust but also stronger and able to communicate more honestly.

In meditation we take this process onto a deeper, more subtle level. We begin to release very deep tension that is held in the way that we think and feel about ourselves and about life. Often we carry around patterns of mental tension from a very young age. Perhaps we think we are stupid, ugly, useless or selfish. Perhaps we think the world is cruel, threatening and unfriendly. Perhaps we think society is an unfeeling machine and we irrelevant cogs in its complex and heartless machinery. All of these ideas create deep, subtle tensions within us that are so much a part of our self-image that we don't even realize it. When we begin to meditate we start to observe these hidden, unconscious assumptions and attitudes. At the same time we observe the patterns of anxiety and tension they create. In seeing this, and the ways that they hurt and impede us, we start to let go: we start to relax about ourselves, about life.

So, gradually and gently, yoga begins to release us from physical, emotional and mental tension. This process can involve many tears and much heartache. However, these are not experienced as threatening or intrusive; quite the reverse. The tears that yoga brings are tears of release, tears of relief. Eventually, as we learn to relax more and more deeply, more and more fully, we learn to live free of the traumas of the past. Then we begin to enjoy the rich beauty of our lives, appreciating the past, enjoying the present and confident in the future.

Yoga is not a movement away from the mundane realm of body, emotion and thought to some higher plane. It is the opposite. It is a penetration of the mundane reality of our life and self-image. It is accepting fully the actuality of our experience of ourself. Through that opening transformation arises: stagnation becomes change, resistance becomes energy, confusion becomes clarity, tension becomes strength, anxiety becomes peace. The great value of yoga is the way in which it can enrich our lives in every way.

One of the most subtle and confusing paradoxes regarding yoga concerns the nature of enlightenment, or freedom. It is not a release from the world; it is not creating a marvellous reality better than our habitual conditioned one; it is not becoming uninterested in the world, our feelings, our minds and entering into a special state of consciousness from which we never wish to return. What yoga gives us is not heaven, but earth; not paradise, but the world; not divinity, but ourselves. We finally let go of all of our psychological clutter – our desires and fears, hopes and ambitions, assumptions and prejudices, preferences and intentions. When we drop these filters we are left with the world as it is. Rain falling wet upon our cheek. The smell of lavender in a hedgerow. The roar of a train in a subway. Rather than adding to them we experience them as they are, in their natural beauty. We experience the outer sensation, the form, and we experience the inner energy, the connectedness. It is a letting go rather than a grasping that leads to a deeper abundance as we become open to the infinite reflected in every finite form.

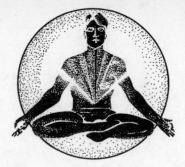

GLOSSARY

Agamas: ancient theoretical and practical treatises on yoga and tantra in particular.

Amrita: the sweet, spiritual nectar that flows from the crown chakra and, permeating the whole body, transforms it.

Ananda: spiritual bliss.

Apana: one of the five winds, or types of prana, that regulate the body's energies.

Arjuna: a mythical prince, the protagonist of the Bhagavad Gita.

Arthava Veda: one of the four main ancient Hindu scriptures.

Asana: yoga posture, the third limb of yoga. A physical position in which stability and comfort can be maintained.

Ashtanga: eight limbs, which constitute the practice of classical yoga.

Aswini mudra: the gesture of a horse, contracting the anal muscles.

Atman: the inner, higher, transcendental self.

Atmanjali: a gesture acknowledging the higher self.

Aum: the vocal expression of the subtle, immanent vibration of the cosmos.

Babaji: an ageless saint reputed to have been living in the Himalayas for hundreds of years in the body of a young man.

Bandha: a muscular grip that has an effect on the subtle energy body.

Bhagavad Gita: one of the major scriptures of Hinduism, the original work specifically on yoga.

Bhakti: the state and process of devotional surrender.

Bindu: a drop, usually of divine fluid or nectar, secreted by the crown chakra.

Brahman: the supreme deity immanent in all creation, or the first god in the Hindu Trinity representing creation.

Chakras: wheels, or subtle energy centres, in the picnic body.
Cit: transcendental consciousness.

Darshana: sight, vision or viewpoint.
Desikachar: contemporary yoga master, son of the late Krishnamacharya.
Dharana: the sixth limb of yoga, mental concentration in which awareness is focused on to a single point, process or activity.
Dhayana: the seventh limb of yoga, in which concentration has become so deep and intense that the mind has become fully absorbed by the object.
Drushti: gaze point, to which the external or internal eye is directed to practise dharana or concentration.

Gheranda: a medieval yoga master.
Gheranda Samhita: a treatise on Hatha Yoga composed by Gheranda.
Gunas: the three fundamental energies or principles of manifestation which underlie and regulate all phenomena: sattva, rajas and tamas.

Hatha: forceful, or sun/moon.
Hatha Yoga Pradipika: a medieval treatise on Hatha Yoga.

Ida: one of the three major subtle energy channels in the body, running around the spine and corresponding to lunar energy.
Ishvara: the Lord, or higher transcendental self.
Iyengar, B. K. S.: contemporary Indian yoga master of international repute, student of Krishnamacharya.

Jalandhara: the net-holding lock, used in pranayama to stimulate the diaphragm and prevent the divine fluid from being consumed by the gastric fire.
Jnana: transcendental wisdom.

Kaivalya: aloneness as a state of liberation from notions and the experience of duality.
Kali: goddess of destruction.
Kapalabhati: cleansing technique for lungs, sinus and brain.
Karma: the process of action and reaction that underlies all activity.

Koshas: the sheaths that constitute the subtle inner bodies.

Krishna: Hindu god, celebrated in the Bhagavad Gita.

Krishnamacharya: late Indian yoga master, teacher of Ashtanga Vinyasa Yoga.

Krishnamurti: late Indian master of meditation and Jnana Yoga.

Kriya: activity, action or process.

Kundalini: the esoteric spiritual energy that lies dormant at the base of the spine to be awoken by yoga techniques.

Mandala: a visual device used for aiding meditation.

Manomayakosha: the inner layer or sheath corresponding to the mind.

Mantra: a special phrase repeated silently or out loud as an aid to meditation.

Matsyendra: regarded as the founder of Hatha Yoga, and mythologically said to have been transformed from a fish having overheard and memorized every word of Siva's teachings on yoga to his consort Parvati.

Maya: the delusive projections of the human mind which distort and obscure direct perception of reality.

Moksha: liberation from delusion and suffering.

Mudra: a gesture, used to recirculate energy and focus the mind.

Mulabandha: the most important technique of Hatha Yoga, Kundalini Yoga and Ashtanga Vinyasa Yoga, by which the anatomical body is stabilized, the nervous system is balanced, the pranic body is harmonized and the kundalini is awakened.

Muladhara: the base chakra deep inside the pelvis, stimulated by mulabandha, which is the seat of the spiritual force of kundalini.

Nadis: the subtle channels of energy which conduct prana.

Nauli: a cleansing technique for the abdominal organs, involving alternating contraction of the abdominal muscles so they appear to be rolling.

Nirvana: the state of release from the cycle of karma, birth and death.

Niyama: the second limb of yoga, involving the application of positive attitudes conducive to the practice of yoga.

Patabhi Jois: a contemporary Indian yoga master, teacher of Ashtanga Vinyasa Yoga, student of Krishnamacharya.

Patanjali: the revered patriarch of yoga, author of the Yoga Sutras.

Pingala: one of the three major subtle energy channels in the body, running around the spine and corresponding to solar energy.

Prakriti: the web of manifestation apparent as the natural world.

Prana: the most subtle energy of manifestation, underlying all other energies and matter; cosmic energy.

Prana: one of the five winds that circulate regulating the body's energies.

Pranayama: the fourth limb of yoga, using the breath to regulate the accumulation and circulation of prana in the body.

Pranidana: total commitment to the spiritual path.

Pratyahara: internalization of awareness, the fifth limb of yoga.

Puraka: inhalation during pranayama.

Purusha: supreme or transcendental self, or pure spirit, analagous to Atman.

Raja: royal.

Rajas: one of the three gunas; the energy or principle of vitality, motion, activity, which in combination with the other gunas constitutes all phenomena.

Ramakrishna: a modern yogi whose disciple Vivekenanda first brought yoga to the West in the late nineteenth century.

Ramana Maharshi: a modern god-intoxicate yogi who lived almost his entire life in a state of ecstatic liberation.

Rechaka: exhalation during pranayama.

Rig Veda: the most well known of the original scriptures of Brahamanic Hinduism.

Sadhana: a committed, consistent practice of yoga.

Sahaja: literally innate or inborn, sahaja samadhi is to awaken and live in the world from a state of ecstatic liberation.

Sama Veda: one of the four original scriptures of ancient Hinduism.

Samadhi: the eighth limb of yoga, the ultimate level of human consciousness with many subtle levels brought about by intense practice of yoga.

Samana: one of the find winds, or organic prana, circulating in the human body.

Samsara: the wheel of birth and death to which we are all bound by the laws of karma until we awaken to our true nature.

Samyama: the process of deep meditation leading from concentration to samadhi, or intense ecstasy; encompasses the sixth, seventh and eighth limbs of yoga.

Sanskrit: the ancient language of Hindu scriptures and yoga texts, which is the source of modern Indo-European languages.

Sat: the state of pure, absolute being.

Sattva: one of the three gunas; the energy or principle of vibrance, luminosity, clarity which in combination with the other gunas constitutes all phenomena.

Shaivaites: devotees of the god Siva.

Shakti: the energetic, female expression of the universe: energy, power.

Siva: the dramatic Hindu god of transformation, energy and destruction, lord of the dance of life.

Siva Samhita: a medieval Hatha Yoga text book.

Sivananda: a modern yogi whose approach to yoga has spread widely in the West.

Sri Aurobindo: a modern yogi, scholar and poet who founded Auroville, a yoga-based community in South India.

Sri Prabupada: the founder of the so-called Hare Krishna movement which has done much to popularize the Bhagavad Gita and Bhakti Yoga in the West.

Sushumna: the most important subtle energy channel (nadi), flowing in three layers up the spine, up which the spiritual force of the kundalini rises through the chakras.

Sutra: a spiritual discourse.

Tamas: one of the three gunas; the energy or principle of solidity, resistance, inertia which in combination with the other gunas constitutes all phenomena.

Tantra: literally a thread, or continuity, tantra is a profound, subtle approach to life and yoga in which all manifestations are regarded as expressions of the divine, and all the natural energies of man and nature are explored, harnessed and transformed for the sake of liberation.

Tantras: texts expounding the theory and practice of tantra.

Tattva: the elements that constitute the natural world.

Trataka: the practice of candle-gazing which develops concentration and strengthens the eyes.

Udana: one of the five winds that circulate, regulating the body's energies.

Uddiyana: the use of the abdominal wall to create stability in the lungs and to stimulate the upward flow of energy.

Ujaiyi: the victorious breath, or the breath of inner fire.

Upanishad: more modern Hindu scriptures.

Vajroli: a subtle, tantric technique for transforming sexual energy.

Vedas: the four ancient Hindu scriptures.

Vinyasa: setting out and returning again, the principle of connectivity, fluidity.

Vishnaivaites: worshippers of Vishnu.

Vishnu: the god of continuity, stability, one of the Hindu trinity.

Vyana: one of the five winds that circulate, regulating the body's energies.

Yajur Veda: one of the four major ancient Hindu scriptures.

Yama: the practice of psychological restraint, the first limb of yoga.

Yantra: a visual device used in meditation.

Yogi, Yogin: one who is devoted to his practice of yoga.

Yogini: one who is devoted to her practice of yoga.

Yuga: a vast aeon of time, of which there are four that make up a single cycle, the mahayuga, covering 1,550,200,000 years, with periods of latency following each active phase.

Dvapara Yuga: an age during which the descent towards the darkness of delusion has furthered itself, lasting 260,000 years.

Kali Yuga: lasting 130,000 years. The current age of ignorance, materialism and destruction.

Satya Yuga: the golden age of enlightenment, lasting 5,200,000 years.

Treta Yuga: an age during which the descent towards the darkness of delusion has begun, lasting 390,000 years.

Zen: the Japanese form of the word dhayana, used to describe a particular approach to Buddhist meditation.

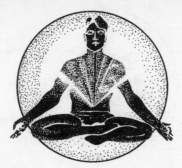

FURTHER READING

CLASSICAL TEXTS

Bhagavad Gita, Penguin, 1970.
Gherandha Samhita, AMS Press, US, reprint of 1914 edition.
Hatha Yoga Pradipika, Aquarian Press, 1992.
Siva Samhita, AMS Press, US, 1992.
The Upanishads, Arcana, 1989.
Yoga Sutras of Patanjali, Sri Satguru Publications, India, 1990.

MODERN WORKS

Bernard, Theos. *Hatha Yoga*, Rider & Company, 1982.
Danielou, Alain. *Yoga, Mastering the Secrets of Matter and the Universe*, Inner Traditions, US, 1992.
Feuerstein, George. *Encyclopedic Dictionary of Yoga*, Allen & Unwin, 1990.
Feuerstein, George. *The Technology of Ecstasy*, Crucible, 1990.
Iyengar, B. K. S. *The Art of Yoga*, Aquarian Press, 1985.
Iyengar, B. K. S. *Light on Yoga*, Aquarian Press, 1990.
Iyengar, B. K. S. *Light on Pranayama*, Aquarian Press, 1992.
Iyengar, B. K. S. *The Tree of Yoga*, Aquarian Press, 1994.
Iyengar, Geeta. *Yoga – a Gem for Women*, Timeless Books, US, 1991.
Narayani and Girish. *The Book of Yoga*, Ebury Press, 1983.
Silva, Mira and Metha, Shyam. *Yoga the Iyengar Way*, Dorling Kindersley, 1990.
Van Lysebeth, Andre. *Pranayama*, Allen & Unwin, 1979.
Worthington, Vivian. *The History of Yoga*, Arcana, 1989.

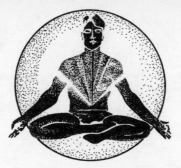

USEFUL ADDRESSES

UK

The Life Centre, 15 Edge Street, London W8 7PM. Telephone: 071 221 4602.

The Iyengar Yoga Institute, 223A Randolph Avenue, London W9 1NL.

The British Wheel of Yoga, 1 Hamilton Place, Boston Road, Sleaford, Lincolnshire NG34 7ES.

USA

B. K. S. Iyengar Yoga National Association of the United States, 8223 West Third Street, Los Angeles, CA 90038.

Richard Freeman 2020 21st Street, Boulder, Colorado 80302. Telephone: 3033 449 6102.

Tim Miller, The Ashtanga Yoga Center, 118 West E Street, Encinitas, CA 92024. Telephone: 619 632 7093.

Thom and Beryl Bender, Hard and Soft Ashtanga Yoga Institute, 325 East 41st Street* 203, New York, NY 10017. Telephone: 212 661 2895.

David Swenson, 1223 Wilshire Boulevard* 639, Santa Monica, CA 90403.

Yoga Works, 1426 Montana Avenue, Los Angeles, CA 90403. Telephone: 310 393 5150.

AUSTRALIA

B. K. S. Iyengar Association of Australia, 1 Rickman Avenue, Mossman 2008, New South Wales.

Graeme Northfield, 44 Tennessee Avenue, Annerley, Queensland 4103. Telephone: 07 892 5800.

Louisa Sear, Mafering Road, Goonengeryy, New South Wales 2482. Telephone: 066 884 097.

NEW ZEALAND

John Scott, 297 Rintoul Street, Berhampore, Wellington. Telephone: 04 389 1181.

Gwendoline Hunt, 15 Creswick Terrace, Wellington.

HOLLAND

Iyengar Yoga Association of Holland, 8 Karthuizersdwars Street, 1015 Amsterdam.

GREECE

The Practice Place, Poste Restante, Agiagalini, Crete.

INDIA

The Practice Place, Bagga Beach, Goa.

BALI

Danny Paradise, c/o Carpenter, Jalang Duyung Gang 1 No. 3X, Semawang, Sanur, Bali, Indonesia.
Telephone and fax: 62 361 287042.

HAWAII

Nancy Gilgoff, PO Box 1001, Makawao, Maui, Hawaii 90768. Telephone: 808 878 2605.

For classes, retreats, book, audio and video tapes by Godfrey Devereux, contact The Life Centre, 15 Edge Street, London W8 7PM. Telephone: 071 221 4602.

INDEX

accomplished pose 102
amrita 56
anatomical body 17, 36, 38
apana 37
ardhachandrasan 86–7
ardhamatsyasan 98
ardhapadmapascimottanasan 89–91
ardhasatvangasan 95
ardhustrasan 93
Arjuna 10
asana 13, 16, 17, 18, 19, 23, 24, 27,
    30, 35, 37, 38, 40, 43–5, 46–7,
    49, 50, 54, 55, 57, 58, 60, 62–3,
    64, 73, 76, 78–103, 104, 105,
    109, 112, 117, 121, 122
Ashtanga Vinyasa Yoga 4, 9, 13, 14,
    16, 22, 23, 24, 61, 63
Ashtanga Yoga 14, 18, 20, 21, 22,
    32
aswini mudra 56, 57, 120
Atman 30, 36
atmanjali mudra 58
attachment 31–2
Aurobindo, Sri 8
awareness body 17

Babaji 24
balance 76
bandhas 17, 19, 38, 54–6, 61
bathing 73
Bhagavad Gita 8, 9, 10, 12, 19, 21
Bhakti Yoga 4, 10, 15, 18, 20–1, 22,
    23, 24
boat pose 92
bound lunge pose 85
Brahman 30, 36, 60
Burmese pose 102

causal body 17, 36
chakras 11, 20, 36, 38–9, 120
chest 74
commitment 42–3
contentment 42, 67
continence 41

dandasan 88–9
Desikachar, T.S. 22, 24, 118
desire 31–2, 34, 41

dharana 18, 21, 40, 48, 50–1
dhayana 18, 21, 32, 34, 48, 51–2
dhayana mudra 58–9
diet 118–20
drushti 17, 59–60

easy pose 102
embryo pose 97
energy 33–5, 36, 44, 46, 59–60, 120
exhalation 106–7, 111, 122
extended triangle pose 86

family life 118
feet 73
folded triangle pose 81–2
folding pose 80
full forward bend 91–2

Gandhi, Mahatma 21
Gherandha Samhita 12, 19, 20
gunas 119

halasan 96
half camel pose 93
half fish pose 98
half lotus cycle 89–91
half moon pose 86–7
half shoulderstand 95
Hatha Yoga 4, 8, 9, 10, 12, 13, 16,
    18, 19–20, 22, 24, 36, 38, 121
Hatha Yoga Pradipika 12, 14, 15,
    19, 20
hero pose 101
honesty 41

ida 17, 38
inhalation 105–6, 111, 122
Iyengar, B. K. S. 8, 22, 23, 118
Iyengar Yoga 23, 61, 77

jalandhara bandha 56, 57, 108
Jesus 25
jnana mudra 57–8
Jnana Yoga 4, 10, 15–16, 18, 23

kaivalya 6
Kali Yuga 16
kapalabahti 61

karma 25–8
Karma Yoga 4, 10, 15, 18, 21–2, 23, 24
karnapidasan 97
Krishna 9, 10, 20
Krishnamacharya 17, 22, 23, 24, 118
Krishnamurti 15, 23
Kriya Yoga 24
kundalini 11, 12, 15, 19, 20, 38, 39, 59, 120
Kundalini Yoga 4, 10, 12, 14, 16, 36, 38, 121

legs 73–4
length of breath 108
lotus posture 102–3
lunge pose 85

mahamudra 57
mandalas 60
Mantra Yoga 22
mantras 22, 60
Matsyendra 9, 23
maya 28–9, 35
meditation 48–54, 59, 60, 109–12, 117, 122
Mohenjo Daro 8
moksha 5, 6, 32
mountain pose 79
mudras 17, 38, 56–9, 111
mula bandha 17, 54–5, 56, 57, 76, 107–8, 120, 121

nadis 11, 19, 36, 37–9
nauli 61
navasan 92
neck 75
nirvana 16, 18, 27
niyama 18, 35, 42–3
non-coveting 41
non-stealing 41
non-violence 41

padmasan 102–3
padottanasan 81–2
Parahamsa Yogananda 24
parsva virabadrasan 82–3
parsvakonasen 85
parsvottanasan 85–6
Parvati 8
parvritasan 94

pascimutan 91–2
Patanjali 9, 10, 18, 22, 23, 53
Pattanbhi Jois, K. 22, 118
pelvis 74
physics 25, 33–4
pingala 17, 38
plough pose 96
Prabupada, Sri 22
prakriti 34
prana 13, 19, 20, 36–8, 45, 50, 54, 73, 104
pranayama 16, 17, 18, 19, 23, 24, 27, 35, 37, 38, 40, 45–6, 46–7, 49, 50, 54, 55, 56, 57, 58, 59, 60, 61, 64, 66, 76, 99, 100, 103–8, 109, 112, 117, 119, 121, 122
pranic body 17
pratyahara 18, 35, 46–7, 50, 59
psychic body 17
puraka 105–6
purity 42
purvottanasan 93

quietness of breath 108

Raja Yoga 11, 12, 13, 15, 18–19, 20, 21, 22, 24
Ramakrishna 15
Ramana Maharshi 15, 23
ramp pose 93
rechaka 106–7
relaxation pose 98–100
resting dog pose 82–3
resting pose 79

sahaja samadhi 32
Sai Baba 23
samadhi 5, 6, 18, 21, 31–2, 35, 48, 52–3
samana 37
samsara 16, 26, 27, 32
samyama 53–4, 57, 112
sanmukhi mudra 46, 59
sarvangasan 97–8
Satyananda 8
savasana 46, 66, 98–100, 104
self-knowledge 43
sex 120–1
shakti 11, 34
shat kriya 60–1
shoulderstand 97–8

sidasan 102
siddhis 20
side fold pose 85–6
side warrior pose 82–3
Siva 9, 20, 60
Siva Samhita 12–13, 19, 20
Sivananda 8, 22, 23–4
Sivananda Yoga 23–4
spine, stretching 101
staff pose 88–9
subtle body 36–9, 54
sukasan 102
supine twist 94
suptaikapadaparvritasan 94
surrender 43
sushumna 38
Svatmarama 12

tadasana 79
Tantra Yoga 4, 11–12, 14, 15,
    16–17, 36, 38, 121
Teresa, Mother 21
Transcendental Meditation 22
trataka 61
triangle pose 81
trikonasan 81
twisting pose 94

udana 37
uddiyana bandha 55, 57, 61, 121
uddiyana mudra 55, 57, 76
ujaiyi 76, 107

union 3–4, 5, 30, 48
Upanishads 8, 10, 12, 15
urdvahastasan 79
uthitta parsvakonassan 85
uthitta trikonasan 86
uttanasan 80

vajroli mudra 56, 57
vasti 61
Vedas 8, 9–10, 12, 15
Vinniyoga 24
virabadrasan 83–4
virasan 101
Vishnu 20, 60
Vishnu mudra 58
Vishnudevananda, Swami 23
visualization 60
vyana 37

warrior pose 83–4

yama 18, 35, 40–1
yantras 60
yoga, effect of 6–7
    goal of 4–6, 30
    meaning of 3–4
    physical benefits of 62–5
    psychological benefits of 65–7
    secular forms of 14
Yoga Sutras 8, 10–11, 12, 14, 18, 19
Yoga Tantras 8, 11–12
Yoga Upanishads 11, 19